DATE			

Raising
Sexually Healthy
Children

Raising Sexually Healthy Children

A LOVING GUIDE FOR PARENTS, TEACHERS, AND CARE-GIVERS

Lynn Leight, R.N., A.A.S.E.C.T.

5478

RAWSON ASSOCIATES : New York

Copyright © 1988 by Lynn Leight
Library of Congress Cataloging in Publication Data

Leight, Lynn.
   Raising sexually healthy children.
   Includes index.
   1. Sex instruction—United States.   2. Parenting—
United States.   3. Parent and child—United States.
4. Sex instruction—United States—Moral and ethical
aspects.   I. Title.
HQ57.L394   1988   649'.65   87-42794
ISBN 0-89256-331-1

Rawson Associates
Macmillan Publishing Company
866 Third Avenue, New York, N.Y. 10022
Collier Macmillan Canada, Inc.

Macmillan books are available at special discounts for bulk purchases
for sales promotions, premiums, fund-raising, or educational use.
For details, please contact:

Special Sales Director
Macmillan Publishing Company
866 Third Avenue
New York, N.Y. 10022

Packaged by Rapid Transcript, a division of March Tenth, Inc.
Composition by Folio Graphics Co., Inc.

Designed by Sheila Lynch

10   9   8   7   6   5   4   3   2   1

Printed in the United States of America

My lover, my best friend, my shield and my sword,
my husband

My loves, my heartstrings, my most challenging blessings,
my children

My nurturers, my role models, my shepherds of spirituality,
my parents

Contents

Foreword

Raising sexually healthy children is the challenge of the 1980s. Everyone wants his or her child to be sexually healthy, but few of us know when and where to begin.

Whether they do it well or badly, parents are the principal sex educators of their children—so they might as well do it well. Silence and evasiveness teach children as persuasively as direct and honest communication. Parents need to appreciate that knowledge is not harmful, but that ignorance and unresolved curiosity *are*. If you are an "askable" parent, your child will begin to ask questions at age three or four or five. Answer them! Tell children a little more than you think they want to know or can understand, thus assuring a perfectly adequate response. (Besides, it's good for children to be exposed to an occasional word they don't quite understand. They'll grow up with an excellent vocabulary.) And relax.

Relax? Easier said than done, you say. You are not comfortable. Let me respond with the confidence of a sex educator who has studied and lectured in this field for more than 35 years. No one is comfortable about his or her sexuality any more (if ever anyone was). No one? Well, almost no one. Join most of us who are not comfortable, but who are endeavoring to become more comfortable. Start by telling your child that you are not comfortable, and your child will reassure you. Then read Lynn Leight's wonderful, warm, compassionate book to better understand your own sexual endowment. This is your unique, family-inspired "golden opportunity" to rehearse the best ways of communicating with your child about anxiety-provoking situations, such as nudity, toilet training, wet dreams, masturbation, and homosexuality. It is the most *au courant* update on teaching your children about safe sex, AIDS, and other vital issues, along with everyday opportunities for discussing sexual health with young people of all ages—toddler to teen.

It's all here—no critical sexual issue is left out. No question remains unanswered. And it's all explained with warmth, deftness, sensitivity, and boldness. When Lynn Leight writes, "A child's sexuality is affirmed or denied at every touch," you feel it deeply, and you know it is true.

Lynn Leight's book presents the alternative we need. When Lynn Leight reveals how a mother calmly handles the "hot" issue of finding her preschooler playing doctor, you laugh and learn by example. When Lynn discloses the secrets shared by a group of eleven-year-olds, you become keenly aware of the sexual curiosity of preadolescents. And when Lynn shares practical resolutions for teens in search of sexual autonomy, you grow wiser and more confident in your role as your child's sexuality educator.

The book is a refreshing view of sexuality with a focus on responsibility, common sense, and spirituality, all in the context of a celebration of family life. A special gift of the book is its final chapter, in which you have a chance to test your new-found information. Dozens of questions and answers provide a treasury of responses to children's most frequently expressed concerns as they mature.

This is the book you wish your parents had read when you were growing up. This is a book you'll share with your friends, your child's grandparents, and one to which you'll refer again and again as your child grows into young adulthood.

Bravo, Lynn Leight!

Sol Gordon, Ph.D.
Professor Emeritus, Syracuse University
author of *Raising Your Child Conservatively in a Sexually Permissive World; When Living Hurts*

Acknowledgments

Four years ago when my dear friend and mentor, Dr. Sol Gordon, advocated that I write a book, a serendipitous chain of events occurred. As if ordained by a higher force, special people and "Golden Opportunities" appeared at strategic intervals to provide guidance and encouragement.

The mission of love began when my secretary, Edith Whittle, typed an abstract on sexuality for a professional journal and enthusiastically proclaimed that I had written the first draft of "The Book." Her influence was so empowering that she infused me with the confidence to submit it to colleagues for comments and review. And so it was Edith's unrelenting faith in the merit of the manuscript and her magical ability to transform hundreds of pencil-scrawled pages into legibly typed print that transformed the dream into a reality.

From the beginning, Judith and Sol Gordon's interest, encouragement, and wise counsel never faltered and will always be appreciated. Dr. Mary Calderone's wisdom and constructive criticism became an influence for which I am greatly indebted. Carol Cassell's delicate and thoughtful review of the original copy and Kathy Everly's technical advice were graciously extended and gratefully embraced. To Judy Rothman (my guardian angel of the publishing world), I offer my deepest gratitude for directing me to Denise Marcil, a literary agent with pluck, judicious intelligence, and a sense of spirituality. Denise helped me choose a fitting and proper publisher with the skill of a professional matchmaker. The reward for such a discriminating selection is an editor such as Toni Sciarra, for whom I have an abiding fondness and deep respect as a consummate professional and a masterful and compassionate practitioner of the written word.

The gossamer thread of serendipity connected me with people too numerous to mention (you know who you are). You will always be lovingly remembered for your direct and indirect contribution in encouraging the completion of this book—persons such as Jody Kay, who proved that an illustration is worth a thousand words, and Jeanne DeQuine, who taught me the nuances of preparing a polished book proposal and techniques for surviving the discipline and pain of editorial revisions. Dear friends who provided emotional and physical sustenance during my self-imposed days in writing exile. Pathfinders of sexual health such as Sid Simon, Michael Carrera, Virginia Satir, Bill Masters, and Virginia Johnson, inspired my perspective of sexuality. Social scientists like Ashley Montague and Norman Cousins, and physicians such as Steve Allen, Jr., and Marty Weisberg who reaffirmed my belief that laughter and humor are the most powerful sources of healing and sexual learning. And my dear, deceased friend, Joan Levy, who was my most ardent cheerleader and loyal supporter. To all who have cared and shared your knowledge and talents and to the countless students, clients, and SHE Center staff who have allowed me to convey their stories . . . thank you. For in truth this book is not *my* book. This book belongs to all of us.

Above all, I wish to take this opportunity to publicly declare my appreciation to my darling husband, my children, and my mother, who have unselfishly encouraged me to complete this project despite the all-night writing vigils, the weeks of isolation, and the months of personal commitment. Certainly my most cherished and sensitive receptors of serendipity have been my family. With their love, support, and incomparable humor, I now know that I can accomplish anything.

Raising
Sexually Healthy
Children

The How-to of Raising Sexually Healthy Children

The sun is just rising on Saturday morning as Stan rolls over in bed to caress his bride of five years. Joanne joyfully responds to Stan's touch. Their bodies are warm and relaxed. The house is peacefully quiet. Stan helps Joanne slip out of her nightgown. Joanne removes Stan's shorts. Stan begins to slide his mouth to Joanne's breasts when he spies—from the corner of his eye—Brian, their four-year-old son, standing transfixed in the doorway.

Stan freezes. His firm erection disappears in a matter of seconds. He rolls off Joanne, controls his anxiety, and greets Brian with a cheery, "Morning, Pal, how you doing today?" With this Joanne gasps and shrills at Brian, "What are you doing out of bed? Go back to bed, *now!* It's too early to be roaming around the house." Brian is in tears as he runs back to his room.

Back in his room, Brian is frightened and confused. He wonders, "What were Mommy and Daddy doing? Why is Mommy so angry? If I'm a bad boy, how come Daddy isn't mad, too?"

This bittersweet incident was the focus of a sexuality seminar I recently conducted. During the past 25 years, I have heard similar scenarios revealed countless times.

One of the greatest joys of conducting sexuality seminars is observing the relief of seminar participants as they discover that they are not alone.

Joanne and Stan's experience opens the door to myriad sexual dilemmas that have afflicted parents for generations: "Once the baby arrives, how can we resume our carefree lovemaking style?" "What happens if our kids catch us 'doing it'?" "If we worry about sexuality now, when our children are only babies, what are we going to do when they are teenagers?" "How can we raise sexually healthy children when we are feeling so confused and guarded and uncomfortable?"

Parents often tell me that they have prepared themselves for childbirth and childrearing on every level *except* for issues related to sexuality. Before attending my seminars on sexuality, many of these parents shunned the subject of sex even between themselves. Too embarrassed to bring up the subject with friends and family, they often feel that everyone else is "adjusting," and that their confusion is a sign of ignorance or sexual inadequacy.

In the safety of the group, each member appears to have a suggestion for Joanne and Stan. I encourage their support. I also remind them that it is always easier to recognize a solution when not actively confronted with a dilemma. In the words of my dear friend and sexuality expert, Dr. Sol Gordon, I caution that "It is easy to be a hero in someone else's shoes."

Some parents keep the bedroom door locked during moments of passion. Some maintain that this isn't always possible, especially if the sexual encounter is spontaneous. Others state that they have never fully enjoyed sex at home since they have had children, knowing that the children are in the next room or down the hall. Some plan their lovemaking when the children are visiting a relative—or they go to a motel and leave the children with a baby-sitter. A very few parents declare that sexual intimacy is a natural expression of deep affection, and that the earlier a child is taught to appreciate this God-given gift, the better adjusted the child will be in the future.

DON'T MISS THE GOLDEN OPPORTUNITIES!

Isn't it a shame that our sophisticated society takes a closed-door approach to such a life-enhancing activity? When pioneers lived in one- and two-room cabins, how were they able to produce such large families without "corrupting" the minds of the children who shared their dwellings? Not that I'm advocating that parents copulate in front of their children (as is done in some societies today), but I doubt that a child will be irrevocably traumatized if he or she suddenly appears during a passionate interlude.

I would classify the situation described earlier *not* as an embarrassment, but as a "Golden Opportunity." Golden Opportunities are the ordinary and extraordinary everyday encounters that can be transformed into spontaneous sexuality learning experiences. Sometimes the opportunity is subtle, like a mother bird teaching her young to fly. Sometimes it is blatant, like a used condom washed ashore in a bed of sea shells. The world abounds with Golden Opportunities. The trick is to grasp the moment as it occurs and address it as nonchalantly as you would any everyday event.

This concept may seem foreign to you if you were brought up with the notion that sexuality education consists of strategically executed "discussions." These discussions usually followed a "crisis": two kindergarteners caught playing doctor, a child found exploring the baby's genitals, or a preteen arriving home late from a date, with her clothes suspiciously wrinkled. Often "the discussion" was a one-time pow-wow reserved for the onset of puberty.

Golden Opportunities, in contrast, are not contrived. They occur at every age and stage of maturation. Within this book, readers will find a treasure trove of Golden Opportunities just waiting to be uncovered. It is this promise of a new, innovative approach to sexuality education that motivates me to write this book.

For years I have helped parents who want to assume their role as their child's primary sexuality teacher, but who don't know how to begin. They fear that they will misinform or, worse, somehow damage their child's sexual health. These parents ask questions like, "When is the right time to talk about sex?" "What happens if I give too much information?" "What if I don't know the answer?" "What if my child doesn't ask?"

Parents are usually surprised when I assure them that *they have been "talking sex" with their child since his or her birth.* Sex talk isn't just about a penis and a vagina. It deals with *every aspect* of life that defines you as a person. Once you embrace this concept, you will recognize that the simple act of washing your child's hair provides a Golden Opportunity to talk about sex.

✳ ✳ ✳ "I love the soft touch of your hair. This shampoo smells so
good and helps your hair shine like golden silk. Did you
know that when you were born you had fuzzy brown hair?
Daddy and I didn't know that all babies grow new hair after
they are born and that it is often different from a baby's first
hair. Hair grows on all different parts of the body. When you
were born, your body was covered with a soft, downy hair,
but it disappeared after a week or so. I guess it shed just like
kitty's hair sheds. As you grow older, new hair will grow on
your body. Just like Mommy and Daddy, hair will grow on
your arms and legs and under your arms and even on your
vulva.

　　Your child may inquire, "What is a vulva?" You
might reply, "The vulva is the name that we call all the
private parts that girls and women can *see* and touch
between their legs." (You may add, "Like the lips of your
vagina, clitoris, and the opening through which you
urinate.") "The hair on the vulva looks and feels different
from your long, silky hair. Now, feel the hair on your arms
and then feel the hair on my arms. See the bristly hair
growing under my arms? Do you want to feel it? Isn't the
body amazing? It's so much fun to talk about how it works
and feels and smells. Hmm, I love the smell of your hair."

　　Now, wasn't that easy! And it really *is* fun when you tune into the
world of wonderment. The prospects are endless. The Golden Opportunity approach has been used successfully by hundreds of parents who
have attended my seminars. It has been trial-tested.

　　If Joanne and Stan had been tuned into Golden Opportunities,
their response to four-year-old Brian might have been:

✳ ✳ ✳ "Oops," says either parent, "you caught us off guard. We
didn't expect company. Mommy and Daddy are kind of
playing with each other. I guess you can call it sex-play. It's
what grown-ups do when they want to show how much they
love one another. It's a special, private time we usually have
together when the door to our bedroom is closed. In the
future when our bedroom door is closed, you will know that

we need private time together. You can knock if you need to ask us something, and we'll tell you if it's OK to come into the room or if the answer to your question can wait until later. If you need private time, you can close your door (don't lock it) and we'll knock before entering, also."

If Brian were your four-year-old son, how would you respond? The sexual dilemmas raised by children and parents in this book will help you recognize that there *is* a suitable solution for every situation.

WHAT THIS BOOK WILL REVEAL

The examples in this book have been gleaned from hundreds of parents and children I have met in seminars and from people whom I have counseled. During the past 30 years, my awareness expanded as my career expanded, first as a nurse, then as a sexuality educator, and now as the founder and director of 16 Sex, Health, Education (SHE) Centers throughout the country. I have been privileged to study with the pioneers of sexuality education, teach sexuality concepts to students from nursery school to medical school, and counsel children and adults in private sessions and through radio, television, and newspapers as well. With every new experience, I have grown wiser. The wisdom is a gift that I share with you. In sharing the techniques that hundreds of parents have used to raise sexually healthy children I have made this book *my* Golden Opportunity to fulfill my life's mission.

I believe that the time has come to rewrite the tired script that for generations has sexually crippled children and adults. With the spiraling number of people seeking sexual therapy, the escalation of reported incidents of sexual abuse, and the consistent prevalence of unplanned pregnancy, new methods to approach sexuality awareness are beginning to be discovered. As parents looking ahead to the increasing danger of AIDS and new strains of sexually transmitted diseases, we see the time has come to legitimize a child's right to know. The question is no longer "Can we talk?" Honest communication about sexuality *is necessary to preserve the health, welfare, and personal happiness of your child.*

Think back. Did you ever walk in on your parents when they were having sex? Or better still: Did your parents ever have sex? Probably not! Sexuality is a subject shrouded with mystery and clouded with misinformation! It is no wonder that we children grew to be adults with little knowledge about how to become our own child's sexuality educator.

TAKING THE SEX OUT OF SEXUALITY

Sex! What is it anyway? How does it differ from sexuality? Most people define sex as intercourse. Others identify sex with being male or female. This book talks about sex, but its major theme is sexuality. Sexuality, as defined in this book, is *the total of who you are, what you believe, what you feel, and how you respond.* It is the way in which you have been acculturated, socialized, and sexualized. It refers to all your relationships and intimate encounters.

Sexuality is all this, including the way in which religion, morals, family, friends, age, body concepts, life goals, and your self-esteem shape your sexual self. It is expressed in the way you speak, smile, stand, sit, dress, dance, laugh, and cry. It defines who you are.

To illustrate this broad concept of sexuality, let me tell you about an adolescent boy who struggles with acne. Every aspect of Steve's sexuality is negatively affected by this condition. He appears aloof and snobbish, shunning social interactions to avoid exposing his self-perceived ugliness. He appears untrustworthy, avoiding eye contact. He walks with a slouch, trying to be inconspicuous, and rarely offers an opinion. He feels too unattractive to dress in the latest styles or wear a pleasant cologne. Steve's unemotional, uncaring facade belies his deep yearning to be touched, to be hugged, and to be kissed.

A smile comes hard to a face that wants to cry. Carried to extremes, teens may deprive their bodies of nourishing food or may overeat, using the added pounds as nurturing insulation or isolation. Alcohol or drug use may mask loneliness and unhappiness. Sexual experimentation or exploitation may be engaged in by a child who seeks affection but lacks the self-respect to use good judgment. It is not his maturing genitals that are shaping Steve's sexuality; it is the acne that undermines his development.

Now that you understand the complexity of the concept, I'm sure that you can think of many examples of situations deeply affecting sexuality: the child who can't measure up to his parents' expectations . . . the young man confined to a wheelchair . . . the woman requiring a mastectomy . . . the man who can't support his family . . . the adult who was abandoned as a child . . . the senior citizen who fears aging.

What is the status of your sexuality? Would you describe it as healthy? Are you pleased with your body? Do you like yourself most of the time? Do you say what you mean and mean what you say? Do you enjoy meeting people? Do you give of yourself and graciously receive from others? Do you value intimacy? Are you willing to forgive? Would you prefer a greeting with a handshake rather than a warm embrace?

It becomes obvious that our sexuality is a lifelong evolutionary process. Throughout this book, you will be asked to think back to your youth so that you may clearly understand your current thoughts and actions related to sexuality.

If you find that certain memories are hurtful, try this exercise to examine the incident with objectivity. Close your eyes and mentally view the incident as you would if you were watching a film. Now take yourself out of the mental image and put a stranger in your place. Concentrate on the action. *You are not in this fictional movie.* The person in the film is someone else. Ask yourself: What is going on here? Who is being used or abused? Who is being misinformed? Who is in control? Who is unhappy? Who is angry?

Decide how this movie could have had a happy ending. Rewrite the plot. Redesign the interaction of the characters. Now, put yourself back in the imagery. Mentally act out the past so that the resolution is exactly as you desire it to be.

It may seem hard to believe, but using this skill, you can reprogram unpleasant memories. Your maturity and intellect will shed a new light on an old perception. A thought is flexible. It can be changed at will. Rethink it with more acceptable resolutions. Next, discard the original thought by letting go or forgiving those involved. Finally, you are free. Now you can move on to gain greater happiness and control over your life.

Penny had been sexually abused as a child. It had been years since she had recalled the unpleasant memory of her baby-sitter's husband pressing her body against his exposed penis while swimming in the family pool. Yet the "film" keeps playing now as she interviews day-care workers for her infant. As much as she wants to pursue her career as a freelance writer, she cannot relinquish the care of her child to another person.

With some skepticism, Penny decides to try my technique for remaking her film. She visualizes a child (not herself) being fondled by a middle-aged man, but she recreates the scene to include an appropriate resolution. The child removes herself from the man's clutches, reveals his behavior to the baby-sitter, and reports the incident to her mother when she arrives home. The caretaker couple is dismissed. The mother reassures the child that she is not at fault, and compliments the child on her good judgment. The child feels safe. She feels good about her ability to distinguish good touching from bad. The mother calls a professional agency and checks the references and credentials of a new care-giver. The mother outlines a protocol for the appropriate care of her child and regularly reviews with the child the day's happenings.

Penny now places herself in the picture. It is no longer disturbing. Penny has changed an old script. How about you? Do you have a sexual script that needs rewriting?

MY PROMISE TO YOU

You have bought this book. That means you *want* to become more sexually aware. You *will* become successful because you *want* to. In the past, sexuality education has been a parenting challenge because parents were simply told the "correct" words to say to their children. No regard was given to the parents' comfort in repeating these words. Feeling inadequate and uncomfortable, parents relinquished their role as their child's sexuality educator. But in today's world, *who is better qualified to educate your children than you?*

- The President of the United States?
- The principal of your child's school?

- Your religious leader?
- Your child's teacher?
- Your child's friends?

This book will help you *and* your children embrace who you are and what you really believe about sex and sexuality. Your children will become emotionally strong as they are assured that all of their feelings are normal. They will grow more confident as they learn that their questions and fears will not be trivialized. It may not always be obvious, but children need and cherish the guidance offered by empathetic and trusted parents. You and your child are natural partners in this journey toward sexual happiness.

THE "COULDS" AND "SHOULDS" OF SEXUAL MORALITY

You may be wondering where morals and ethics fit into the scheme of this sexual journey? Actually, you can't discuss sex without talking about morals. Where do morals come from? And how do they affect our sexuality?

Let's define morals and ethics as guidelines that help us distinguish between what is right and what is wrong. Morals may differ depending on the dictates of a person's religion, culture, or government. I believe that we practice two kinds of morals. One set of morals is what we should do and the other set is what people actually do. You may have heard a person say, "I don't believe in abortion, but if I became pregnant, I guess I'd have one." Because morals are subject to change, they may be confusing.

It's the "should" aspect of morals that is the most sexually damaging. "Should" is a word that sets up standards that usually are in conflict with our actions. In defying this "perfect" set of values, a person often feels guilty. As a general rule, I sidestep the "shoulds" that constantly emerge in my life. "Should" can tyrannize our belief system. "You should always respect your elders" and "Children should be seen and not heard" are examples of beliefs that may actually place a child's safety in jeopardy, since a child who is socialized to respect *all* adults indiscriminately may be more vulnerable to sexual abuse.

Warren has spent his entire life doing exactly what his father told him he "should" do. He hates the profession and lifestyle his dad dictated he "should" pursue. The contempt he feels for himself is evidenced in his inability to form an intimate relationship. Warren is impotent—a sexual metaphor for his powerlessness in life. At age 32, Warren asks, "Is it possible to break the 'should' habit?"

Yes! Even a lifetime of conditioning can be reversed. Whenever I counsel with someone who is held captive by "shoulds," I'm reminded of the giant circus elephant obediently confined by a single rope casually looped over a wooden stake. Certainly, the elephant has the power to break free. After all, outside of captivity, elephants uproot trees. But the elephant has been conditioned since birth to believe that it *should* obey the restrictions of the rope. The elephant is so tyrannized by what it *should* not do that *it does not even know that it can be free.*

I propose that the word "should" be removed from the vocabulary and replaced with "could." When you do this, you are freed from what you believe others want you to do and you can act upon what *you* believe. For example, one modern ethical dilemma is whether or not to tell a potential sexual partner that you have herpes. You may say, "I really should." I may ask, "Who says so?" You may shrug, "I don't know. I guess that most people would think I should." "But," I ask, "what do *you* think?" Now rephrase the question, replacing "should" with "could." "Could you tell your partner?" "Could" implies that you are acting in accordance with your own belief system. It is hoped that you will say yes because *you* believe it is ethically correct.

Morality and ethics are crucial in molding sexuality. Babies are born amoral. For the first two years of life, they are concerned only with having their needs met. Between the ages of two to seven, they begin to have a notion of what rules are, even though they change them to satisfy their desires. Often the endless "why" questions asked by young children are really "how" questions. "Why is her tummy big?" is really "How did she get pregnant?" The true "why" questions are the ones that have moral content. They are answered early in life:

- Because it is unkind
- Because it is hurtful
- Because it is unfair
- Because it is dishonest

These simple answers lay the foundation for the deep ethical issues connected to sexuality. Your sensitivity to your child's questions proclaims your "askability." It encourages the child on his or her path to seek the truth. Between the ages of 7 and 12, children rigidly abide by certain rules of society imposed upon them by the adults in their world. Soon after, however, they begin to show a deeper grasp of right and wrong by questioning moral and ethical issues. As teens, their moral judgments shift often and quickly, especially in the face of peer pressure. The more knowledge and social interaction children have, the better able they will be to make responsible sexual decisions. With their maturity comes the sensitivity to the sanctity of each person's body, social priorities, self-worth, and rights. What a beautiful gift you can give them!

This is why it is a disservice to our children merely to hand down moral absolutes. It is certainly not wrong that there be "absolutes," but each of us must choose his or her *own* code of absolutes from a thoughtful analysis of the choices and the probable consequences.

As the primary agent of sexual information, you have three choices: You can parrot responses dictated by the so-called "sexperts." You can repeat the messages from home that have molded your own sexuality, or you can develop an eye and an ear and a sensitive soul to recognize Golden Opportunities for creative learning. It begins with the loving, natural interplay of a child reaching out and a parent warmly responding.

I encourage you to hold fast to the values that best define your belief system and to improve your effectiveness as a communicator by trying to see things from a child's point of view. As you read on, the basic concepts of how to do this will become clearer.

I believe that in all of life there is a master plan and a fine gossamer thread that connects us, not by chance, but by choice. The Hebrews refer to this predestined path as *barshert*. The time is right for us to meet. I'm excited by the power that we share to transform sexual silence into sexual enlightenment. With the knowledge gleaned from this book, your children will be able to move ahead without the vulnerability that accompanies sexual ignorance. This knowledge will become the core of their confidence and will safeguard them against exploitation and disappointment. Knowledge is the most precious endowment that we can give to our children. It is the legacy that you give them and *their* offspring as you continue your quest to raise sexually healthy children.

2

Valuing Your Values

During my 30 years of marriage, I have revised the personal value system that I adopted as a child. Our three grown children have influenced my values, as have my friends, clients, and colleagues. The evolution of a person's sexuality is a lifelong process. It is affected by experience and knowledge, and may also be influenced by the political, economic, social, and cultural environments in which we move. Values change as people change. Values are neither right nor wrong; they simply are a fact of life. By looking at your values, you are able to uncover your true, often hidden, feelings about sex.

WHERE DO YOU STAND ON SEXUALITY?

I ask that you pause now to answer on a separate sheet of paper the questionnaire provided here. There are no correct answers to this self-test. It is your barometer to help you understand your beliefs and see specifically the values you are transmitting to your children. If your life-style does not meet your values, you will have a clearer idea of the areas that need to be brought into harmony. You may wish to share this questionnaire with your partner or a close friend. It's always enlightening to see how differently people feel about the same sexual issue. The questionnaire is a great way to open avenues of stimulating conversation with friends and family. You may find discussing it more fun than playing charades when the party gets dull!

While the statements are divided roughly into social, cultural, and religious areas of influence, it is important to recognize that these influences cannot be neatly separated. For example, as a social consequence you may believe that masturbation is a healthy outlet for a widow or widower, but from an ethical point of view you may not approve of it for married couples.

Ethically, you may approve of masturbation for others, but your personal belief that the genitals are unclean may dissuade you from partaking of the activity. You may approve of masturbation for others but disapprove of it for yourself, if you believe that it defies the laws of the Bible. Or you may not agree with the biblical denouncement of masturbation, but culturally you believe it is an acceptable activity for men only. Then again, you may have embraced the Bible's injunction against masturbation, but you may have modified this belief in light of the political edict encouraging masturbation as an alternative to intercourse and the risk of contracting AIDS.

You may approve of the medical merits of breast-feeding your baby. Socially, you may be influenced by the current trend to breast-feed, as well. Culturally, breast-feeding may be endorsed as the ultimate symbol of maternal love. In addition, you agree that breast-feeding provides many practical and economic benefits. However, you dislike the concept because of some vague fear of its sexual connotation and your concern that it may have a negative influence on your ability to resume your sexual responsiveness to your husband. Or you feel it will delay your return to full-time work away from home.

To complicate matters, myths—masquerading as truths—have shaped the sexual belief system of generations. Untold thousands of women have become pregnant believing that they couldn't conceive the first time they had sex. Men have dreaded the promise of insanity as a result of masturbation. People have avoided public restrooms believing that gonorrhea is spread from toilet seats. The list of myths is endless.

This questionnaire is a personal inquiry that endorses your right to affirm or denounce a belief. The important issue is that yesterday's truth may not be today's. And today's values may not hold true tomorrow.

QUESTIONNAIRE

Where Do You Stand on Sexuality?

Rate your response to the following statements using the scale below.

5	4	3	2	1
Strongly agree	Agree	Undecided	Disagree	Strongly disagree

1. A mother is a child's best sex educator.
2. In a single-parent household, a child has a more difficult time understanding sexuality.
3. It's a woman's job to keep her man satisfied, regardless of her desires.
4. Men have a stronger sex drive than women.
5. The man should be the aggressor in lovemaking.
6. It isn't healthy to allow your children to see you undressed.
7. It's OK for kids to see their parents argue.
8. It's unhealthy to let boys play with dolls.
9. A mother's love is natural and instinctive.
10. A man who doesn't have intercourse before marriage is either a wimp or gay.
11. Real men do not diaper babies.
12. A child should be encouraged to explore his or her body.
13. When children play doctor with one another, it's time to separate the sexes.
14. Sex is so confusing for me. I'm afraid I'll pass my confusion on to my children and they won't grow up to be sexually healthy.
15. Too much holding will spoil a child.
16. A father is the best sex educator for a boy and a mother is best for a girl.
17. Breast-feeding is not sexy.
18. It's embarrassing when your child takes forever to be potty trained.

19. It's not healthy for a father to hug and kiss his children in public.
20. A child should be punished for using "dirty" words.
21. When referring to body parts, it's better to use words children understand, like "peepee," instead of confusing them with anatomical terms.
22. A person with a sexually transmitted disease probably sleeps around a lot.
23. A naked body is ugly.
24. Most men are afraid of strong, competent women.
25. Girls need to be held more than boys.
26. Sexy people are those who are attractive and have a great body.
27. Cologne and deodorant must be used to avoid offensive body odor.
28. A parent is entitled to privacy, but a child is too young to appreciate its value.
29. I can live without sex; it's more trouble than it's worth.
30. Sometimes my sexual urge is so strong that it scares me.
31. If I don't know the answer to a sexual question, my child will not respect me.
32. Mothers who place their infants in day-care centers are shirking their responsibility.
33. Girls should be dressed in soft, frilly pastels.
34. You shouldn't bathe children of the opposite sex together.
35. I masturbate because it's healthy and pleasurable.
36. Raising a child is a science. In order to do it well, you must rely on the experts.
37. Every time we talk about sex we have an argument, so I avoid the subject.
38. As often as I try to change, I keep repeating the same mistakes my parents made when I was a child.
39. Being a parent means feeling guilty most of the time.
40. It's OK to lie to a child if it saves him or her from pain.
41. You need not tell your partner you have herpes if you have no active lesions.
42. It's OK for teens to have sex if they use condoms.
43. Divorce is never the right answer.

44. Children aren't ready for sexuality education until they can verbalize their questions.
45. Sex education does not belong in the schools.
46. Reading stories about sex or looking at pictures of sex acts is perverted.
47. Homosexuals should not be permitted to teach in the schools.
48. No one, other than me, has the right to talk to my children about sex.
49. When a woman has her period, she is unclean.
50. The more information you give a child about sex, the more curious he or she will become.
51. If a person is irresponsible enough to get pregnant, she should not penalize the baby by getting an abortion.
52. It's OK for my boyfriend to sleep with me, if he leaves before the children wake in the morning.
53. I can't enjoy sex without love.
54. My parents did the best job they were capable of doing when it came to sex education.
55. Good parents sacrifice their sexual desires to satisfy their child's needs.
56. It's only fair that my husband share equally in raising the baby.
57. God intended intercourse for procreation.
58. Good children do not masturbate; it is against the Bible's teaching.
59. The church is best equipped to teach sex education.
60. Morality does not change.
61. If you follow the codes of your religion, you need not feel guilty about sex or anything else.
62. Neither women nor men should have intercourse until after they are married.
63. In a religious home, the man is the boss.
64. Abortion is wrong under any circumstances.
65. If you train your children in God's laws, they will not stray from your principles.
66. When you provide your children with absolute values, they are less likely to make unwise choices.
67. Homosexuality is unnatural and deviant.

68. Virginity is the best gift a woman can give to a man.
69. Living together without being married is sinful.
70. A person may be a loyal follower of his or her faith without upholding all of its teachings.
71. It's abnormal to have sexual dreams or fantasies.
72. AIDS is a punishment for those who practice amoral and promiscuous sex.
73. Just when I think I have a grasp on my sexuality, I hear a sermon and I feel guilty again.
74. Homosexuals should not be accepted as church members.
75. Sexual sinners can be redeemed if they commit themselves to God's path.

How did you do? Were there value-laden issues that challenged your sexual frame of reference? Was there a "Yes!" or "No!" response that begged a "but" as an addendum to your initial reply: "Yes, a mother is a child's best sex educator . . . but in some instances perhaps a teacher, counselor, or father may be better equipped to provide first-hand information." "No, it is not healthy to allow your children to see you undressed! . . . but it can become a valuable teachable moment when the time and circumstances are compatible with a parents' comfort level." "Yes, virginity is the best gift a woman can give a man . . . but what if the woman discovers, after marriage, that she and her husband are sexually incompatible?" "No, I don't masturbate! . . . but if I could get over my dislike of touching my genitals, perhaps I would try."

If more questions were raised than resolved, then you are on the right track for discovering greater sexual enlightenment.

After you complete this book, I recommend that you take the questionnaire again. Since most of these issues will be discussed in the chapters that follow, you will have an opportunity to confirm or reject your current point of view. Remember, seeking the truth is a lifelong process. Your inquisitiveness will become a valuable asset as you embark on the sexual awareness journey with your child.

3

A Baby Is Born

Robin, at 25, and Mike, at 27, have learned through the magic of ultrasonography that in two months they will become the proud parents of a healthy son. While Robin is happy, she is concerned that she will "make a mess of raising a boy. My parents were divorced when I was nine," she tells me. I grew up with Mom, Grandma, and my younger sister. I never even saw a penis, other than Mike's."

"I'm not exactly an expert on raising boys, either," Mike reveals. "I was raised in a family of all girls." In recalling their sex education, Robin remembers, "Most of my learning happened one summer when I went to camp, and of course, I learned a lot from Mike." Mike never remembers speaking to either of his parents about sex. He learned everything from "friends, movies, and 'on-the-job training.' "

Robin and Mike are determined to make their parenting career a success. Together, we began to look at the earliest and frequently unrecognized messages that set the tone for a child's sexuality.

THE JOURNEY BEGINS

I never felt as close to miracles as I did when I worked as a labor and delivery nurse. I clearly recall the sanctity of the moment when a newborn, still bathed in its amniotic fluids, is gently placed on its mother's abdomen. This extraordinary being is totally unlike any other child yet born or ever to be born. He or she has a customized thumbprint that says, "I'm Thumbody. I'm the first, the last, the original!"

19

The birth of a baby completes an incredible nine-month engagement, which sprang from the improbable meeting of one egg out of an ovarian storehouse of approximately 400,000 eggs-in-waiting. Only one sperm, from several million candidates, will be "approved" by the egg and accepted for fertilization. The attraction must have been ordained to overcome the one-in-three-hundred-trillion chance that they would meet and like each other. In the moment of conception, the potential human receives its genetic dowry of every trait that it will ever own.

It takes the dividing and combining of more than 70 trillion cells before a new human being emerges from its mother's body. The umbilical cord is severed. No longer an amphibian receiving blood and oxygen through its placenta, the baby gasps its first breath. In that instant, the newborn claims full status as a uniquely designed human being, born with the desire to receive love and the potential to express it.

BONDING: TO HAVE AND TO HOLD

From its first moments in the world, a baby begins its lifelong search for security and identity. Every reponse of its caregivers molds its perspective.

Within the first month, this tiny social being seems to sense when it is not wanted. It is acutely aware of the signals, like a shrill voice, rigid body, or cold, unsmiling face. Love and trust evolve as the baby begins to see that its needs are consistently met. The first need, believed by many to be the most important predictor of a baby's sexual adjustment, is the need to suck. Sucking, be it from the breast or the bottle, along with being cuddled, *prepares the infant to give and take intimacy in its adult life.* In infancy, love means having one's needs met. In adulthood, mature love is the delight in meeting the needs of another.

The mother–child bond is believed to be the crucial aspect of a child's development, especially during the first six months of life.

Even now, as we celebrate the wonderful bond between children and the increasing numbers of father nurturers, modern research still corroborates that mothers, by way of biology or by cultural/social programming, continue to have the most profound influence on a child's earliest perception of love, intimacy, and relationships. I believe, however, that the studies have not withstood the test of time. It may take another generation before research can document the impact of the distinct nurturing style of men. It is estimated that by 1990, 80 percent of mothers with toddlers and infants under the age of three will be working outside the home. As parenting styles change to adjust to mother and baby's needs, nurture and nature will adjust to our new social norms. What we do know for sure is that the male parenting figure is an important partner of the "nurturing team."

SEX ROLES: OH BOY, IT'S A GIRL!

Few of us can remember the early years of life, so it is hard to realize that *it is during this period of our lives that the sexual script by which we will express ourselves as adults is being written.* Regardless of background, each of us assumed a conditioned sex role from the moment we were assigned a name. With that name came expectations, as parents dreamed and planned for the future.

For generations these expectations have been colored blue for the aggressor, while the nursery of the pacifist, the receptor, and the nurturer has been colored pink. From the moment of birth, parents literally and figuratively color their expectations according to the baby's sex.

For centuries, boys have been told never to take "No" for an answer as preparation for their role in life to achieve and succeed. As men, they applied the same dictate to relationships, assuming their prescribed role of sexual dominance. A girl was told to pacify and cajole as preparation to entice a man who would bring happiness and security. As a woman, she was conditioned to assume her role of sexual submissiveness. As a teen, she was told to say "No" to hormones that encouraged her to say "Yes" to premarital sex. But on her wedding night, she was to say "Yes" to the sexual desires she had suppressed.

If you are a mother or mother-to-be, perhaps you were programmed to believe that the role of a daughter was to:

- Grow up just like Mom.
- Be neat, be clean, be soft, be sweet-smelling.
- Master female skills: cooking, teaching, nurturing.
- Be pretty, be popular.
- Assert feelings, but not opinions.
- Be warm, be gentle, be yielding.
- Maintain a good reputation. In time, the message may have been: Good girls . . . don't.

And what was said to sons?

- Be a jock, like Dad.
- Be objective, be logical, be analytical.
- Be independent and adventurous.
- Be powerful, be competitive, be ambitious.
- Be successful.
- Keep a stiff upper lip.
- Never take "No" for an answer. In time, the message was reinforced with: Real boys . . . do.

What childhood messages have conditioned *your* sexual belief system?

- Boys are always capable of doing better.
- Girls must not exceed their limitations.
- Boys are natural athletes and professionals.
- Girls forfeit their femininity if they pursue athletics or a professional career.
- Boys must be conditioned for acqustion and conquest.
- Girls must be socialized for appeasement and compromise.

Nicole is now 38. She has been in psychotherapy for one year. Nicole's soft, sweet voice, delicate features, and slight figure belie her age. She has been married for 20 years and is the mother of two teenage boys. Nicole had to undergo psychotherapy as a prerequisite for her graduation from a master's degree program in counseling. The requirement has dramatically changed her life. For the first time, she is addressing issues from her youth that have been buried and unrecognized.

Nicole remembers the day her baby brother was brought home from the hospital. The moment he arrived, she felt abandoned. He was her mother's prince and Dad's big boy. Whatever Dad's boy wanted, he got, including a college education, which was not on Dad's agenda for sweet, petite Nicole. At 18, Nicole married a clothing salesman ten years her senior. Whenever Nicole talked about starting school, her husband had an economic crisis that compelled her to withdraw. Then came the children—two boys.

Well," Nicole smiled, "I guess you are wondering why I'm here and how I managed to enter graduate school. Ten years ago, I stated that either I was going to enter college or I would leave my husband and children. My demand was triggered by a simple incident that brought me right back to my youth. Our oldest son received a partial scholarship to go to summer camp. For the first time in my life, I *raged*. I was mentally reliving an incident from the past when our family was awarded a scholarship to send one of us to camp. I was the oldest; I deserved to go." Nicole's voice grew bolder and more aggressive. "But no, my brother was selected to go, because 'boys need the experience of a competitive athletic challenge.' This time, years later, I decided that *I* would come first."

For the 11 years since Nicole entered college, she has sexually withdrawn from her husband. She has given him license to get sex whenever and wherever he pleases. Somehow the arrangement has worked. Now, as Nicole begins to understand the hostility she harbors for all men, including her sons, she is beginning to reconsider those negative feelings. In therapy, we worked to help her establish a healthier opinion of herself as a valuable person in each of her roles as professional, wife, and mother. She is beginning to accept that she does not have to annihilate her sexuality in order to achieve her goals and that she need not forfeit her femininity to claim opportunities for self-fulfillment.

Recently, in a parent sexuality seminar, we were discussing the subtle factors that perpetuate sex stereotyping. From children's fairy tales to adult literature, men are still portrayed as clever and resourceful, independent, and competent. Girls continue to be portrayed, but with less frequency, as compliant and dependent, more fearful and less competent than boys. As we talked, Paul leafed through his photo album, which is the required "text" for my seminars. (This unorthodox "text" is a thoughtful chronicle of photographs from infancy to the present date. The "text" helps a parent remember the childhood events that have subtly shaped his or her sexual belief system. The "text" also helps parents recall experiences and emotions that help them understand their children's needs.)

Paul paused at a birthday party photo taken in 1957. The photo pictured children in party hats. All the boys were swashbuckling pirates; the girls were helpless damsels in distress.

Years have passed and the party guests are now adults. Perhaps one of these party guests has reappeared as an able-bodied Prince Charming to awaken and rescue the frail Sleeping Beauty and sweep her into a sexual encounter. One hopes that Prince Charming also was a Boy Scout and remembered the motto "Be prepared."

And what of the damsel? Women who have forfeited their assertiveness and competence in the hope of being "rescued" by fairy tale heroes take a risk that their horses will be turned back into mice and their coaches into pumpkins. The larger risk is that a woman abandons her self-esteem, while a hero's untimely death or divorce may leave her as pathetic as Cinderella in search of her slipper.

Sexual stereotyping is so deeply rooted that liberation is a constant struggle. Yet I have counseled many Prince Charmings who have confessed that they are tired of pretending, tired of fulfilling another's fantasy. Often they feel scared, ignorant, and inept, and have great difficulty expressing or receiving tenderness. The damsels confide that they feel emotionally and sexually bankrupt. They are afraid to trust another "hero." Both run from intimacy, fearing the burdens of an emotional entrapment.

As adults, you have the opportunity to introduce *modern-day heroes and heroines* to your children. Develop a distrust of books and games that glorify computers for boys and clothing designs for girls. Include in your reading biographies of Amelia Earhart, Eleanor Roosevelt, Golda Meir, and Susan B. Anthony, as well as the traditional male heroes.

Of course, the most important role model is *you*. Through example children learn that it is okay for Dad to cook dinner and Mom to balance the checkbook. It is perfectly acceptable for Mom to buy flowers for Dad and for Dad to surprise Mom with new photographic equipment. Mom and Dad can steal a kiss with equal enthusiasm, as well as express an interest in football, art, economics, and lovemaking. These sexuality lessons are just as easy to teach as social skills such as "please" and "thank you" or safety rules such as "cross on green" and "don't accept candy from strangers."

What sex stereotypes were you taught in your youth that you still cling to today? These stereotypes may express themselves in the name you select for your baby, in the color you choose to paint the nursery, and in the clothes and toys with which you surround your child.

WHAT'S IN A NAME?

An exercise that I find to be revealing is to ask clients how they feel about their name. Candy hated her name. "For as long as I can remember, people have made wisecracks about how sweet I must be. Now that I'm an adult, I realize the constant sexual pressures I have been put under because of my name.

Jim hated being called "Junior." "I always felt that I had to live up to the expectations of Dad, Jim Senior. Even now, as an adult, I believe that I won't allow myself to succeed because it may embarrass Dad if I'm more successful than he is. The worst part about being called Junior is that it makes me feel like a little boy. Little boys aren't supposed to be sexual turn-ons."

Henrietta wished that she had fulfilled her parents' dream to have a son. For her whole life she has been called Hank. "It's impossible to feel feminine with a name like Hank, so I never tried. I wonder how different my life would have been if my name were Debbie or Gloria."

You may resist the idea of bucking sex stereotypes. It takes a concerted effort to bypass the eyelet and lace, even when you know that denim is the more practical purchase for your petite, rosy-cheeked daughter. It may take considerable soul searching to question the merits of calling your son "Junior" when you desire that your son grow up to be his own person, not a carbon copy of the past generation.

Family and friends may challenge your decision to abandon pink for red, claiming that such subtle influences will not assist baby girls to grow into corporate executives. Grandparents may insist that the world isn't ready for aggressive women and that tenderness is not a male virtue. Try to be sensitive and patient. We are all fledglings in attempting to turn the tide of the limitations placed upon both sexes. Explain that today the changing world is providing more opportunities to people who dare to be soft *and* aggressive, competitive *and* compassionate.

BREAKING THE PERFORMANCE HABIT

Even with our heightened awareness of sex-typed behavior, it continues to be encouraged. Research shows that mothers cuddle girls more often for a longer period of time and for more years than they cuddle boys. Parents talk more tenderly to girls. Fathers jostle infant sons in play, but handle daughters with loving care. A girl's needs are often responded to with dispatch, as though she were more fragile and helpless than a boy. A daughter's tears are more likely to tug at the heartstrings, while a boy may be told, "Big boys don't cry. Come on, be a man."

Is it any wonder that grown men so often struggle to relate with empathy and warmth, while grown women often complain that their spouses don't seem to care?

A woman of 24 seeks counseling. She has been married for only six months, but she wants a divorce. "It won't work," she tells me. "He's unresponsive to my needs. He's too stoic, too macho." Before they were married, she had been fascinated by his cool, mysterious facade. She thought that marriage's intimacy would reveal his emotional side. It didn't. Now his silence is frightening to her: "I can't make love to a stranger."

Too often, boys are taught to suppress their terror of failure in their mission to succeed, to keep their "eye on the ball" and "back to the helm." A man may become so accustomed to manipulating people to reach his own ends that he must later struggle to bring honesty to any relationship. The performance habit may become so urgent that it expresses itself even in the intimacy of the bedroom. The haunting demand to "do it better" or "be the best" may sabotage a man's control of his ejaculatory response. Alternatively, the specter of failure may become so frightening that he is unable to achieve an erection at all. The need to prove competence undermines a man's ability to admit his human need to be held, coddled, and consoled. The inability to risk exposing their emotions, fears, and doubts may account for the high degree of depression, loneliness, and even suicide among aging men.

Girls, on the other hand, are permitted to cry but forbidden to fight. They grow into adults who subdue and fear their anger. This makes them vulnerable to abuse and open to exploitation. Girls learn at an early age that tears can be one of their greatest allies.

Tears are a way of persuading without fighting. Often, a tearful young woman can get her way with a man who is otherwise an immutable force. These same tears hinder a woman's ability to establish an honest, mature relationship. Frequently she feels unappreciated and unloved when her partner cannot decode the specific concerns hidden by her veil of tears. Her unmet emotional needs may lead to suppressed anger, which evidences itself in more tears, as well as diminished desire for sexual sharing.

WHAT AM I FEELING?
COMMUNICATING EMOTIONS

When parents encourage children of both sexes to display the *full range* of emotions, including anger, fear, loneliness, depression, confusion, and doubt, as well as happiness and joy, they are preparing their children to become ethical, assertive, clear communicators. There'll be no game-playing or second-guessing in their children's relationships, because emotions will be available for discussion. These children will protect one another's dignity as they mature into sexually healthy adults.

One method that will help you and your family to express

emotions is simply to ask yourself: "What am I feeling?" It sounds so simple, but few people actually stop in the middle of their busy lives to ask this question. The range of feelings is endless: joy, despair, anger, happiness, appreciation, love, confusion, fear, doubt, shame, frustration. Once you have identified your feeling, you may answer the question, "I feel angry or happy or sad because _____."

One caution: If you find yourself changing the statement to: "I feel that . . ." you are no longer expressing a feeling. You are making an objective observation; you are actually expressing a thought, not a feeling.

For example, six-year-old Larry continues to use inappropriate language, even though you have explained to him that such talk is not acceptable. You say, "Larry, I feel angry when you ignore my request to stop using this language." The message is clear that you are angry. If you had said, "I think *that* (or I feel *that*) you ignore my request not to use this language just to get me angry," you are conveying an observation that may or may not be correct. It doesn't affirm that you are angry (and you *are* angry!). It also insinuates that Larry is purposely manipulating your emotions. If the assumption is false, you owe Larry an apology for assuming he's guilty of a crime he didn't commit. You may also be setting Larry up to fulfill your accusations in the future. This is what's known as a self-fulfilling prophecy. The only fact that you know to be true is that you're angry. That is the emotional reaction that will be helpful for Larry to understand.

Marsha and Frank are concerned about Esther, their three-year-old daughter. They describe Esther as a quiet, passive child. Now, with the new baby at home, Esther is even more noncommunicative. "She's hard to read," Marsha says. "Half the time I don't know if she says what she means or if she means what she says." Frank laughingly adds, "She's just like her mother. She says one thing, but her body language and facial expressions say something else. Often I don't know if my wife wants to be close to me or not. Like Esther, my wife sends out mixed messages."

Marsha was raised in a tumultuous household with highly emotional parents. Marsha learned to repress her emotions out of fear, or as she prefers to call it, "respect." Now she is modeling this behavior to her daughter, and it is hampering the family's relationships. That's sad. But Marsha is pleased that the family has identified the problem and that there are solutions.

The next week Marsha joyfully reported that she had transformed an everyday occurrence into a Golden Opportunity:

✳ ✳ ✳ Three-year-old Esther was moping around the house. Marsha asked Esther how she was feeling, to which Esther shrugged and said, "I don't know." "Are you feeling sad?" Marsha asked. "Are you feeling angry? Are you feeling happy?" Again Esther shrugged. Marsha said, "Come, let's find out how you are feeling."

Marsha led Esther in front of a full-length mirror and asked softly, "How is the girl in the mirror feeling?" At first Esther just made a funny face. Before long, however, both Marsha and Esther were laughing into the mirror, creating an array of faces and movements that portrayed a given emotion. Together they showed one another what disappointment looks like and how embarrassment looks different from sadness. Esther loved the game and later spent hours coaxing the baby to make a happy face in the mirror. Marsha also learned a lot about herself. "You know," she told me, "I never realized that when I say 'Yes' I often shake my head as though I mean 'No.'"

A few weeks later, Marsha announced that Esther and Frank had created another Golden Opportunity. While flipping through a magazine, Esther stopped at an advertisement for acne cream and pointed to the model in the ad, saying, "Look Mom, she looks sad." When she turned to a toothpaste ad, she exclaimed, "This lady is happy!"

Together, the family created an ingenious barometer for measuring one another's emotions. They posted an assortment of faces, cut out from magazine ads, each depicting a different mood, onto a piece of cardboard. The faces ranged from "Very Happy" to "Very Sad," with an assortment of other feelings such as tired, mean, and angry. The plan was to place a sticker next to the face that best described each person's mood for the day. In just a few months, the family had improved their emotional connection a hundredfold, and Esther was learning how to be expressive in her relationships.

SELF-ESTEEM IS A SEXY SUBJECT

Self-esteem and its link to sexuality may not be immediately understood. Yet whenever I attend a sexuality seminar in which teenage pregnancy, sexual exploitation, and dysfunction are discussed, self-esteem is prescribed as the single most effective panacea. The people there all nod their heads in affirmation while I wonder, but where do you get high self-esteem? How is it developed? If you don't own it, where can you buy it? And what is it, anyway?

Self-esteem is your idea of who you are and your opinion about how the world views you. It is influenced by myriad factors. Just when you think it is intact, a new challenge tests its durability. As an infant, it is having one's needs met. It is learning to trust. As a toddler, it is appreciating the functions and individuality of the female or male body. To the preschooler, it is relinquishing the natural romantic attachment for the parent of the opposite sex. (This will be explained in more detail in later chapters.) To the school-age child, it's learning to be independent by expanding social and intellectual skills. To the adolescent, it is blending monumental hormonal surges, body changes, sexual urges, academic expectations, social pressures, and separation from parents. To a young adult, it is choosing a career and making decisions about finding a marriage partner and raising a family.

THE SELF-ESTEEM SCRIPT

Hi! I'm self-esteem. I trust my family and friends. I value my beliefs. I have faith in myself. I appreciate being a girl or a boy, and I like the traits that define my masculinity and femininity.

I accept the expectations and limitations of being male or female. I understand that I, like everyone else, have strengths and weaknesses. I feel secure in my parents' love. I acknowledge goodness in others. I'm open, optimistic, and adventurous. I predicate my success on my abilities, wit, intellect, physical appearance, and convictions. I have a "can do" attitude and realistic goals. I accept responsibility for my actions. There is a consistency to my life.

You can spot me in a crowd. When I smile, people respond because they like me. When I talk, people listen because they respect me. When I laugh, it's from joy, not because of the hardships of others. When I cry, it's to help me cope with disappointments, frustrations, and sadness. I use food to nourish my body. I use touch to nourish my skin. Communication nourishes intimacy, and lovemaking nourishes my libido.

Caring for myself and the rights of others is my way of nourishing my soul. Achievements nourish my spirit. Every part of me is beautiful. I am confident without being conceited. I'm somebody special and, no matter what happens, I believe in myself.

You say you want the self-esteem script for your child? It begins at birth. Every expression, touch, and caress is a message that shapes your baby's self-esteem. Self-esteem is nurtured by the number of positive experiences a child has during the formative years. It springs from the way each achievement is greeted. The first step, the first word, the first use of a spoon, no matter how awkward, are but a few events that call for praise and recognition. Praise is in order for learning how to dress, tie shoes, comb hair, and a host of other milestones. These early lessons may not seem related to raising sexually healthy children, but trust me, they are vitally important! Here are two Golden Opportunities that can happen with little ones:

✳ ✳ ✳Daniel takes his first step. Dad is there to applaud the accomplishment. Later in the day, Daniel is encouraged to demonstrate his new skill to the rest of the family. The achievement is greeted with exclamations of joy: "Hurrah for Daniel!" Daniel loves being the center of attention. He recognizes that he is being appreciated. Daniel now has the incentive to take two steps, then three, and finally to walk with confidence and run with pride.

❊ ❊ ❊Sara attempts to comb her hair by herself. Mother controls
her impulse to take charge as Sara tries to unsnarl the
tangles and place a part in her hair. Mother sits on her hands
while Sarah awkwardly adjusts a ribbon in her less than
perfectly coiffed hairdo. Sara looks in the mirror and smiles
with pleasure. Mother now has the option to recomb Sara's
hair or to accept enthusiastically Sara's first attempt as a
glorious achievement. If her mother praises Sara's success
without any reservations, Sara will gain greater independence, pride in her appearance, and confidence in her skills.

Eventually the messages sent by smiles and praises are internalized, and
a child begins to believe in himself or herself. As teens and adults, they
will not give their hearts or bodies to others in an attempt to win the
affirmation and love that should be a part of their sense of self.

ASSAULT AND REPAIR OF SELF-ESTEEM

Throughout our lives our self-esteem is assaulted. Remember giving up
Mommy's lap so that she could breast-feed the baby? Remember
getting separated from your parents in a department store? Remember
falling down, causing your team to lose the relay race? Remember being
the first one to misspell a word in the spelling bee? Remember being the
smallest/tallest/fattest/thinnest/smartest/dumbest kid in your class?
Remember being rejected for membership in a school club? Remember
being stood up for a date? Somehow you survived. How did you repair
your wounded ego?

It can be difficult to recognize how and why self-perception
falters. Three children may share the same parents. Two appear to be
self-satisfied. Yet one child rarely smiles, has few friends, and appears to
have a low opinion of herself. Why? I don't know! The parents don't
know either. One child may perceive a compliment as a threat to future
accomplishments, while another may use it as fuel for future successes.
That is not to say that the parents should feel as though they have failed.
It *is* to say that building one's sense of self-esteem is a tricky business and
that the foundation is laid early in a youngster's life. A child's self-
perception may be influenced by sibling rivalry, a parent's illness, or a

change in the economic and social structure of the family and many other factors beyond our control. The consequences, however, are *not* irrevocable.

One woman told me, "I've got hang-ups. Who hasn't? My parents did the best they could. But there was something inside me that kept fighting their efforts to make me feel good about myself. If they told me I looked pretty, I didn't believe them. If they *didn't* tell me I looked good, I'd worry that I must look horrible. As I got older, I decided that I wasn't the prettiest, but that I wasn't ugly, either. It was then that I realized that it's *me* who has to convince me that I'm OK. That's when I began to be kind to myself. Every day I would give myself a compliment. When I said it, I believed it. And so I said it over and over again.

"I have taken charge of my hang-ups. When I was unable to have an orgasm, I didn't have the money for therapy to discover the childhood events that were causing me to hold back. So I started to liberate myself in different ways. I splurged on a new hairdo—because I deserved it. I risked asking for a raise—and got it! I pampered myself with herbal baths. And I bought myself a subliminal cassette tape that I listened to every day. The simple message that was muted by the sound of the music kept repeating, "Relax—you can have an orgasm. You deserve it. You owe it to yourself." I had little faith in the tape at first. In fact, I felt stupid buying it. After all, it was like my parents telling me I was pretty. But after a month, I began to repeat the message to myself. And within weeks my "me" began to believe me. Voila! I had my first orgasm!

"Now, as a mother, I make a point of complimenting my children every day—even if they wrinkle their noses in disbelief. Sometimes I write with lipstick or toothpaste on the mirror so that when they wake in the morning they are greeted with 'Hi, sunshine, your humor cheers the day' or 'Good morning, handsome, you have a great smile.' I slip notes in their lunch bag to remind them of how much they are loved or to cheer them on: 'You'll pass the test. You studied hard and you deserve to pass.' I don't wait for a special occasion to buy them a small gift or bake their favorite dish just to say 'I love you.' Whenever I have the chance, I remind them of their greatness. I'm convinced we can do whatever we really want to do, and what is undone we choose not to accomplish. Two of my kids already believe it. The other two are working on it."

Through the years parents have shared with me a wide variety of Golden Opportunities for enhancing their child's self-esteem. Some of the ideas seem far removed from sexuality, but now you can appreciate the far-reaching value of encouraging children to *make informed choices, assume responsibility, and take charge of their lives.*

Here are two creative Golden Opportunities:

✳ ✳ ✳After being enlightened to my Golden Opportunity theory, Caroline initiated a self-esteem-building idea for her 18-month-old daughter. Rachael was the focus of the family's affection, and was catered to like a princess. But after learning about the virtues of self-esteem, Caroline realized that effusive love is not necessarily healthy love. The family agreed that a real gift of love would be to help Rachael, at this tender age, to become a responsible family member. Eye-level shelves were built in Rachael's room to store her toys. Simple drawings of the toys were painted on the backdrop of the shelves to help Rachael locate the appropriate space to store her playthings. The shelves were topped with a bright yellow sign with red letters: "Rachael's Toys." Family members demonstrated how to stack, pile, and store the toys. In time, Rachael took over. She was applauded for removing and replacing her things. She was encouraged to choose freely any toy for play. She was complimented for assuming the responsibility for cleaning up her own things. Rachael, at 20 months, was taking pride in her competence and in her ability to take care of what belonged to her.

✳ ✳ ✳Joshua and Enid, two parents in the sexuality group, embraced the self-esteem concept even before their son Jamie was born. From the moment of birth, Joshua chronicled, by means of a video camera, Jamie's history. The "firsts" were recorded: the first step, the first haircut. The "favorites" also were recorded: the favorite toy, the favorite food. Videotapes of special occasions and celebrations were preserved for posterity and shown to Jamie as he grew up. As a consequence, at an early age Jamie had a clear self-concept. He was able to:

- View himself as others see him
- Hear himself as others hear him
- Describe his own body language and facial expressions
- Watch his body change and grow
- Relive celebrations
- Document achievements
- Affirm strengths and uniqueness
- Accept weaknesses
- Laugh at shortcomings
- Reconfirm trusted friends and loving relationships

Of all the Golden Opportunities for raising sexually healthy children, I cannot think of a more ideal concept than making you and your children the stars of your own family production!

4

Touch Is a Touchy Subject

To touch and be touched is probably the most crucial aspect of sexual health. From the moment of birth, the skin transmits to the infant the feeling of safety, caring, comfort, trust, and love. The skin is the body's uninterrupted sensual wrapping, containing infinite numbers of pleasure centers. *A child's sexuality is affirmed or denied with every touch.*

THE POWER OF TOUCH

Almost everyone can remember the irresistible urge to touch the velvety skin of a newborn baby. A mother in our sexuality group told of her birthing experience: "Labor isn't fun. I was angry at everyone—my childbirth coach, the doctor, my husband, and even my not-yet-born baby. But the moment the doctor placed my squalling baby on my abdomen, I was filled with the most incredible sense of joy. I'll never forget the silky, slippery touch of my baby's skin. I hadn't planned on breast-feeding, but I changed my mind when I realized the sensual ecstasy of holding my baby to my breast."

Whether a baby is breast-fed or bottle-fed, the skin-to-skin cuddling that accompanies the experience is thought by many theorists to be more vital than the milk itself. Many studies have shown that newborns who are deprived of the nurturing touch do not thrive. Babies who are cuddled tend to be more content; they sleep better and are more responsive. Touching enhances a baby's intellectual and physical growth.

36

The need to be touched throughout life takes different forms, but is never diminished.

- The child crawls onto a parent's lap.
- The preschooler cuddles a fuzzy toy animal.
- The teen participates in contact sports.
- The football player pats his teammate's rear end.
- The adult enjoys an intimate embrace.
- The senior citizen strokes the cat curled on her knee.

At some point in most children's lives, however, touching becomes infrequent and hugging becomes awkward. When this happens, children usually find substitutes, satisfying the need to be touched by roughhousing with one another or accidentally bumping into each other. Many children grow to adulthood starving for skin nourishment, and too many adults can barely recall the last time they kissed or embraced their parents.

If you doubt the power of touch, pause a moment and gently cup your left arm with your right hand. Slowly caress your forearm, your elbow, your biceps, and the inner crease where your elbow bends. Now, stop! How does your left arm feel? Is it warm and comforted? How does your right arm feel? Is it cool and neglected?

Imagine how soothing a back rub can be to a child who is raging from some frustration. Imagine the emotional nourishment you can provide your child by gently caressing his or her arms or legs or back while you both watch television.

Despite the proven virtues of touching, many adults refrain for fear of encouraging inappropriate behavior or erotic fantasy between child and parent. I would like to reassure these parents that everyone, at one time or another, has had a strong desire upon which they have *not* acted. The fact that the parent is fearful is an indication that she or he has the ability to control these urges.

In a healthy person, these urges are fleeting and self-controlled. There are times when I crave ice cream. The urge becomes stronger and my mouth waters as I fantasize about the refreshing, sweet flavor.

I may even say that I'd give "anything" for ice cream. But ice cream is an unacceptable treat on my diet. I am committed to following my dietary rules. I may choose a substitute for my craving, like sweetened iced coffee, or I might change my focus of attention to my work, a book, or TV. Erotic urges that are off limits are just as easily, if not *more* easily, controlled than any other pleasure urge.

I encourage you to relax and enjoy the pleasure of a nurturing touch with your children. Nurturing touch is provided by gently massaging or caressing any part of the body *except* the places that are sexual by nature, the genitals and surrounding area. A nurturing touch may be an embrace around the shoulder or waist, a neck rub, ruffling someone's hair, or a body hug that is as warm and snuggly as a fur coat.

GUIDELINES FOR COMFORTABLE TOUCH

With the increasing number of divorces, a new "touchy concern" has arisen. Stepparents have confided that they restrain their natural inclination to display affection for fear of appearing seductive. I have even heard adults confess that they wouldn't consider remarriage until the children are grown. "You know," they say, "stepparents are often tempted and are more tempting than biological parents."

For those who are concerned about a new parent joining the family, I suggest that you and your future spouse rehearse a conversation that may be shared with the children.

"David and I love each other and will soon be married. David also loves you and would like your permission to show you how much he cares about you. He would like to kiss you good morning and good night and invites you to do the same. David enjoys putting his arm on your shoulder in public. He says that it makes him feel proud to protect you and show the world that he loves you. At times, David may like to kiss you or hold your hand in public, too. How do you feel about David's request? David wants to talk to you personally, but I thought you and I should talk first so that you have time to decide what will be best for you. Remember though, if at any time you feel uncomfortable with the way you are being touched, tickled, hugged, or kissed by David—or me or anyone else—you must say, 'No, I don't like that' and then tell me right away. It's important for me to know that no one makes you feel bothered, embarrassed, bad, or sad.

"Above all, if someone does something that makes you feel funny and asks you to keep it a secret or wants to give you a gift to keep the secret, tell Mommy right away, because it's important for me to know. You won't get in trouble. You'll just get a big hug and kiss from me."

In light of the recent publicity concerning child sexual abuse, we can't afford to deny the possibility that our children may be coerced or exploited by an adult or adolescent. The fact is that, in 80 to 90 percent of the reported cases, the offender is someone the child loves and trusts. And while the most common time for sexual abuse to begin is between the ages of 3 and 11, it is never too early to educate children to the sanctity of their body. On the other hand, it is equally important that children not be intimidated into interpreting every innocent touch as a threat to their safety. It is vital that children not become fearful of all touch. They need to recognize that there are many people who are safe and can be trusted. Remember that speaking in absolutes without regard to the *nature* of the touch and the *person providing* the touch may have negative consequences for the future.

✳ ✳ ✳ Bath time offers a wonderful Golden Opportunity for sensitizing baby to sensual pleasures, as well as introducing children to discussions about the wonders of the body. Sponges, soap, bubbles, and water toys add to the joy of the bath. Using words like "warm," "cold," "soft," "slippery," and "Mmm, good," Mom or Dad increases baby's sensual awareness. In this playful atmosphere, Mom or Dad, referring to each part of the body by its proper name while it is being washed, initiates the correct "body language." In time, children will repeat the correct terminology as they take charge of washing their calves, navel, elbows, penis or vulva, and between their toes. Children can be tenderly instructed as to which body parts are most sensitive to gentle care, as well as cautioned to the dangers of inserting objects into ears, eyes, anus, vagina, nose, or navel.

Bath time allows parents to alert children to the parts of the body that may be exposed and touched in public (all parts not covered by a bathing suit) and the private parts of the body that remain covered and are not to be touched (penis, vulva, anus, buttocks) by anyone except the child and Mommy, Daddy (or Nana, Aunt Jean, Dr. Hicks). Bath time allows children to take charge of their bodies, as well as reminding them that you are a trusted friend to whom they can report if another person exceeds the boundaries of safe touching. After the bath is a wonderful time to gently rub baby's body and massage baby's skin with creamy skin lotion. Phrases like "Mmm, smells so good" and "Oh, so pretty," accompanied with positive, loving facial expressions, not only fulfill your child's need for skin nourishment, but also reaffirm the beauty of his or her body.

TOUCH AND THE NURSING MOTHER

Touch as a touchy subject often arises in our parent sexuality group. "For months after I stopped nursing the baby, I froze when my breasts were touched in lovemaking." "It took me nearly a year to transform the nurturing feelings I associated with my nipples and my breasts to the erotic feelings of having them kissed and fondled." Many mothers have found that while nursing or bottle-feeding, sensual pleasures may at times escalate to sexual feelings that make them feel uncomfortable or guilty. Mothers often suppress these feelings. I assure these mothers that as normal, sensuous beings it is only natural that skin-to-skin contact may trigger a sexual response. The same holds true for the baby, who may be aroused to an orgasm in response to the pleasure achieved from the oral sucking reflex.

All human beings are born with their sexual system intact. Male erections have been viewed in utero by means of ultrasonography and, while the same phenomenon for girls is difficult to document in utero, research has ascertained that infant girls may also experience an oral orgasm, at which time their vagina becomes moist and the clitoris may become slightly enlarged.

As I share this information with you, I can imagine the dismay of some readers to whom the thought of an infant having a reflexive orgasm is unacceptable. Please rest assured that if and when it occurs, the parent is not at fault. The baby is not at fault. The response is no different than a sneeze. The body is only doing what comes naturally.

We are all capable, from the moment of birth, of experiencing erotic pleasure from many sources of stimulation—from the warmth of the sun to the pulsating rhythm of a hand-held water massager. If only we could accept the inherent naturalness of our sexual system as we do the digestive and elimination system, we would be well on our way to raising sexually healthy children.

BOUNDARIES FOR TOUCH

I have always been a "toucher." When I talk, my hands automatically reach out to personalize our discussions. I curb this reflex action when I sense that it makes a person uncomfortable. We all have an invisible bubble that defines our parameters for closeness.

Through the years, I have learned to ask permission to invade that bubble. I might say, "I'm so happy for you, I'd like to hug you." I never take a rejection personally. What I have found is that at first people accommodate my expressive touch with some reserve. In a short time, however, warmth and trust are established, and they, too, are reaching out.

Studies have found that appropriate touch has a positive effect on every species. The librarian who touches the hand of a book borrower is likely to increase the borrower's respect for the library. The teacher who touches a child's shoulder will encourage the student to satisfy the class requirements. The kitten who is patted will purr with contentment. The lover who is stroked will become a more responsive partner.

Through touch, a parent can help a child to be assertive about what kind of touch is acceptable, as in the following Golden Opportunity.

✳ ✳ ✳ Father and four-year-old daughter are sitting in front of the television. Dad puts an arm around the child's shoulder and absentmindedly allows his hand to rest on his daughter's undeveloped breast. Daughter assertively says, "Daddy, you're not supposed to touch my breasts. It's a 'private part.'" Daddy smiles with approval. "You're right, sweetheart. I'm sorry. I guess I was not thinking. I'll be more careful." Dad removes his arm and asks his daughter if she'd like a massage. Daughter joyfully accepts the invitation. Father says, "I'll rub your legs, your toes, your arms, your fingers, and your back. Is that OK?" Daughter says, "OK, but will you rub my neck and scalp, too?"

Daughter has been educated since infancy as to which parts of her body are "private." She knows that all the parts Daddy mentioned are OK because they are "public" parts that are not covered by a bathing suit. Dad reassured daughter that she could relax to the pleasure of massage by listing the body parts he intends to touch. He did not ridicule or embarrass her for requesting that he remove his hand from her breast. Dad also showed daughter that he didn't feel rejected or insulted. In fact, he rewarded daughter by offering her the gift of a massage on her terms. Dad's desire to be affectionate was met, and daughter's desire to be safely touched by Dad was fulfilled. Everyone is a winner!

SELF-TOUCH

As I open the discussion on self-touch in a parent sexuality seminar, one parent calls our attention to his "text." We laugh in response to a photograph of a gloriously happy nude child sitting in a bathtub. You can almost hear his squeals of joy. "Look where his hands are!" the father laughingly challenges the group. "Wouldn't you be happy if you knew it was OK to put your hands there!" With that, I ask the group to close their eyes and try to recapture their earliest memories about masturbation. As quiet concentration envelops the group, I prod their memory.

- Do you remember what you were told?
- Were you admonished, "That's bad! Don't touch"?
- Did you set the family in a state of frenzy by touching yourself in public?
- Were your hands or your genitals gently slapped?

- Were your hands abruptly removed?
- Were you reminded of the church's prohibition?
- Did you begin to develop a sense of guilt every time your hands followed their natural inclination?

One parent opens the discussion with a personal confession, which brings tears to her eyes. "All my life I have hated my vagina. I could never understand how my husband could be aroused by me. When the doctor took me off birth control pills and fitted me for a diaphragm, I knew there was no way that I would ever use it. Not if it meant touching *that place*."

She pauses and smiles. "That's how Scott was born." Then she continues. "Counseling has helped me understand the origin of my problem. My mother hated sex, and she was also a cleanliness nut. Before going to bed, I always had to bathe. After the bath, I showered to remove the grime that the bathwater supposedly had left on my body. My mother had special brown washcloths that were only to be used to wash the 'dirty parts.' Often she would wake me from sleep because I had rolled on my stomach and my hands were tucked under my thighs, near my vagina. When I awoke, I was not permitted to touch anything until my hands were washed. I remember wondering as a child why the big fuss about washing my hands. How dirty could they be? It took me forty-two years to learn that my body was not dirty and untouchable. What a waste—what a damn waste."

Natalie's story is a variation of a theme that I have heard many times: the man who as a child was whipped when his father discovered him masturbating and who now won't get a vasectomy because the after-care requires that he masturbate in order to ascertain that his ejaculate is sperm-free . . . the young woman who was taught that she should never touch her "nasty" and wears a panty liner every day to protect her lovely lingerie from her dirty vagina . . . the young man who won't use a condom because he's been taught that it's dangerous to handle his penis.

Babies are born without any sexual inhibitions. By age six months, they have explored all their cavities and appendages. The body invites the infant to become a friend to all its parts. A baby will find its genitals and discover that this feels good, too. And why not? It is one of the baby's pleasure zones. The baby owns it and has every right to claim its pleasure potential.

By 18 months, the baby already knows which touching is considered appropriate and inappropriate. The parent imparts this message by facial expressions and voice tone. When negative body language is consistent with the sharp verbal command, "No, no," the baby begins to be conditioned effectively to believe that the genitals are not to be touched. If the parent considered the nose to be an undesirable organ of the body, the same rules of negative conditioning would be equally effective. The infant would mature into adulthood with the fear and anxiety that he or she would inadvertantly sneeze in public. If, God forbid, he or she did sneeze, the guilt associated with wiping his or her nose might require a lifetime of psychotherapy to resolve!

Parents who have grown to understand the value of genital play will convey a different message to the baby. When daughter coos and smiles as she touches her vulva, these parents respond with a smile of acknowledgment and "Yes, sweetie, it feels good." If their infant son happens to have an erection, be it from self-touch, a gentle touch when a parent powders the baby or a response to the cool temperature of the room, the parents will not panic, turn their eyes away, or throw a diaper over the penis (except perhaps to deflect a urine spray). The parent will affirm that it's OK with a warm smile and words of affirmation: "It's OK, old chum. It happens to the best of us." By 24 months or older, as a child's intellectual abilities grow, the sexually comfortable adult can reaffirm that "Yes, touching yourself should and does feel good, doesn't it?"

Sigmund Freud, who explained human behavior in terms of one's sexual energy (libido), claimed that all children around the age of four instinctively and naturally acknowledge their gender and the pleasurable sensation they derive from touching their genitals. If children are deprived of this developmental curiosity, Freud postulated that the prognosis for becoming a sexually healthy adult is reduced. Most sexologists and social scientists agree with Freud's conclusion and endorse masturbation as a natural, healthy aspect of one's sexual unfolding. In fact, in an effort to remove the taboos associated with masturbation (which literally means to mutilate oneself), modern terminology, such as "self-pleasuring," was developed to connote pleasure and natural inquisitiveness.

Whether or not we choose to acknowledge it, we all have masturbated in our lifetime. Remember the good feelings evoked from rubbing the genital area against the side of a chair or rhythmically constricting the thighs? These pleasurable spots or erogenous zones may differ from person to person and may have been blocked by negative conditioning.

Jill told the sexuality group how she dealt with her four-year-old daughter's habit of pleasuring herself at the "wrong times and in the wrong places." Jill prefaced what she identifies as a Golden Opportunity with a little personal history: "It took a lot of self-talk and gentle persuasion from the group and my husband to convince me that it wouldn't harm the children to acknowledge the naturalness of genital play. Whenever our daughter played with her genitals, I took a deep breath and smiled affirmatively, even though my stomach was in knots. After a while, though, when I saw how content and well-adjusted our daughter was, I became more convinced that I was doing the right thing. The only problem now is that she's so comfortable with self-pleasuring that she does it whenever and wherever she pleases! I've wanted to discuss with her the necessity of choosing the right time and the right place, but I couldn't find the right words to talk about it until the other day when I uncovered a Golden Opportunity.

✳ ✳ ✳ We had just finished her bath and she had water trapped in her ear that refused to be coaxed free. I gently rotated a cotton swab in her ear and in a moment the water was absorbed. "Mmm," she said, "that feels *tingly*. Can you do it some more?" Again, I gently swabbed her ear. She was in ecstasy. Then she asked if she could do it to herself. Aha, I thought, our sexy little four-year-old has discovered another pleasure zone. Here at last was my Golden Opportunity. I asked, "Can you think of another part of your body that makes you feel this good when it is touched?" "No," she replied. "Think real hard," I said. "Isn't there a part of your body that makes you feel tingly when you touch it?"

She smiled and pointed to her vulva (external genitalia). "Well," I continued, "your ears are like your vulva in that they both feel good when they are touched. But you can't swab your ears, just like you can't rub your vulva, *all* the time, because it will become sore or irritated if touched too much. And you can't put just *anything* inside your ear or your vulva because it is tender and it can be bruised easily. Also, you can't clean your ears or play with your vulva *anytime* you want because people will think you are being rude. Can you imagine how silly you would look if you swabbed your ears at the dinner table or in the grocery store?" We both laughed. "Well," I continued, "swabbing your ears is only to be done occasionally, with gentle care, in the privacy of the bedroom or bathroom." I cautioned her about the safety factor of inserting a pencil or toothpick in her ear and vagina, as well. "I'm glad you got water trapped in your ear today because it gave me a chance to talk to you about touching private parts of your body in private places like your bedroom. If you should forget, I will remind you by saying 'private please,' and you will know that is our secret message that means that this is a public place and please wait until you have privacy." We both agreed that the plan was good. I can't tell you how relieved I felt! At long last I had confronted the subject and neither one of us was embarrassed. Hurray for me!

One last note about genital play. I am often asked, "How much is too much?" A couple expressed their concern that their five-year-old son Barry is obsessed with touching his penis. Whenever he is left alone, watching television or playing quiet games, he rubs himself until the area becomes irritated and sore. This type of compulsive behavior, like all compulsive behavior, may be a sign of an emotional disturbance.

Perhaps Barry feels that the new baby has usurped his place of importance. He may feel neglected and in need of warmth and affection. He may be displaying hostility in the form of hurting or punishing himself because Mommy, for whom he has a strong attachment at this age, is preoccupied with the new baby. Perhaps he senses the anxiety he is causing Mommy and Daddy, and wants to exercise his power and his control: power to do as he pleases, control over the act itself and the family harmony.

Together, we planned a program for improving the quality of time that Barry shares with his family. Mom and Dad are to make a concerted effort to satisfy Barry's need for skin nourishment with back rubs and foot massages, and at least three hugs a day from each parent—real body hugs that say "I love you." Exclusive time each day will be set aside for Barry and a parent to do anything that Barry pleases. It was suggested that the time include experiences like assembling a puzzle or baking a cake, where there would be opportunities to share feelings and thoughts, and assure Barry that he is still a star in the expanding family. Certain special toys are to be kept in reserve for times when Barry appears bored and neither parent is able to give him undivided attention. As for the obsessive behavior, all nagging, threats, bribes, and demands concerning it are to be eliminated.

Mom and Dad were challenged to find a Golden Opportunity to discuss their concern about obsessive behavior at a time *unrelated* to the activity. Otherwise, they agreed to ignore the behavior unless it continued to take place in public places. In that case, Barry would be directed to pleasure himself in his bedroom. Two days later, Mom stumbled on a Golden Opportunity:

✳ ✳ ✳Mom and Barry had used their private time together to bake brownies. As they were measuring the ingredients, Barry had the bright idea of adding three cups of sugar instead of the prescribed two cups. Mom asked Barry what he thought would happen if an extra cup of sugar were added. He said, "The brownies will taste better because they will be sweeter." Mom suggested that they follow the recipe exactly as written for one batch of brownies, but that a small portion of the batter be reserved for additional sugar. The outcome was that Barry hated the brownies with the extra sugar. "Yuck, they're terrible! They're too sweet!" he exclaimed. Mom was now ready to proceed with her Golden Opportunity. "You see," she said, "too much of a good thing is not always so good. There are lots of things in life that are only good in small amounts. Flowers love sun, but when they get too much sun, they don't do so well. Fish love their food, but they can get sick if we feed them too much. These brownies are delicious with just the right amount of sugar, but they get icky when you add too much sugar. It's kind of like when you pleasure yourself. At first it feels nice and that is good. But when you rub too much and your penis gets sore, it's not pleasurable anymore. It's important not to overdo any good thing so that it doesn't lose its specialness. Next time you stroke your penis, just think about the brownies."

The idea of self-touch may be in conflict with the beliefs with which you were raised. As you rethink how you stand on these values, please consider some of the facts. Research has disclosed that self-pleasuring:

- Promotes a child's acceptance of his or her sexuality
- Increases a child's sense of sexual identity
- Becomes a legitimate substitute for premature sexual encounter
- Expands a person's range of sexual expression (outercourse as opposed to intercourse)
- Avoids the hazards of contracting sexually transmitted disease, especially AIDS
- Allows people to understand how they are best fulfilled sexually
- Offers opportunity to convey personal knowledge of sexual fulfillment to a partner
- Expands options for the safer, barrier forms of birth control that require self-touch, such as the diaphragm, sponge, and condom
- Promotes responsible sexual health care through self-examination
- Provides a healthy, appropriate way to relieve sexual tension (especially for adults when there is no partner available and for persons of all ages choosing abstinence)
- Enhances responsiveness and orgasmic ability in both men and women

Despite all the evidence in favor of self-pleasuring, you may be grappling with the emotional tapes from your childhood of parents' admonishing that such behavior is wrong or sick. Perhaps you were told that people who masturbate will become homosexuals and that the activity will destroy their ability to enjoy sexual arousal with a person of the opposite sex.

If you are stuck between fact and fiction, intellect and emotion, past and present, I urge you not to feel pressured to decide which "truth" you now hold to be self-evident. For you this may be an area that will require more thought and more discussion. Reserve your opinion until you reach the last chapter of this book, when you will be invited to answer the questionnaire from Chapter 2 again and take a new inventory of your values.

5

Preschool Sexual Dilemmas

The parent sexuality group has selected preschool sexuality dilemmas as the subject for discussion. The comments and questions come fast and furiously: "When should we stop undressing in front of our two-year-old son?" "Help! I found our five-year-old son and his three-year-old cousin half-dressed playing doctor in his bedroom." "My husband is convinced that our seven-year-old son wants to become a girl." "Our four-year-old is so busy playing that I don't know how or when to introduce the subject of sex." I put a cap on the questions and promise to answer them all today.

POTTY TRAINING: A GIFT OF LOVE

Barbara and her husband have a child sexuality caper that she just can't wait to tell. Their major project for the past six months has been to entice two-and-a-half-year-old Timothy to move out of diapers and onto the potty seat. For the past few weeks, Barbara and Tim eagerly raced to the potty every time he made a grunting sound and gestured to his genitals. Since most of the potty drills turned out to be false alarms, Barbara no longer accompanied him to the bathroom, but cheered him on as he did his bathroom dash.

Barbara relays yesterday's incident. "I was on the phone as Tim grunted, pointed, and streaked to the bathroom. I cheered him on as usual and continued my conversation. I could hear Tim clapping his hands and reciting some nursery rhyme. He sounded OK, but just to be certain, I put the call on hold and checked it out.

"When I looked in the bathroom, I didn't know whether to

laugh or cry. There was Tim, as happy as a lark. Yes, he had made a bowel movement in the potty, but then he had *retrieved* it and was using it to make handprints on the bathroom walls, gleefully reciting 'pat-a-cake, pat-a-cake.' "

Barbara was surprised, but far less unnerved than she would have been if she had not been a member of our parent sexuality seminar. She no longer gave negative messages by grimacing at the sight of Tim's soiled diapers and even laughed when Tim's stream of urine went astray, using the moment as an educational opportunity for acceptable bathroom decorum. Barbara was aware that children often express their pleasure in their ability to take charge of *all* of their body's processes in the form of examining their spoils.

Barbara couldn't resist laughing as she looked at Tim's smudged face. He looked like a devilish clown exuding whimsy. Without thinking, she joyfully hugged Tim. As they went about cleaning up, Barbara explained that while she was proud of Tim's success on the potty, she was not happy about the clean-up task. "A bowel movement," Barbara said, "is like chewed-up food. *The food is good, but it's not nice or polite to take the food from your mouth and play with it at the table.* When you play with your food, your hands get sticky. That's why you wipe your hands with a napkin and wash them with soap and water. When you make a bowel movement and you play with it, your hands get sticky and messy, too. And just like you wipe your hands after you eat, you always wipe your anus after you make a bowel movement. And, to make sure your hands are clean and there are no germs on them to get into your mouth, you always wash your hands before leaving the bathroom, just as we are doing now. This is how you will stay healthy and feel comfortable, too." (Notice that Barbara avoided such negative words as "filthy," "dirty," "bad," and "disgusting." She also provided Tim with as much information as she felt he was able to handle. If she offered more than he could understand, that's OK; she would repeat it again, clarifying the information as Tim's comprehension abilities increased.)

Barbara may later expand the details of the food's journey from ingestion to elimination. Since children's learning is enhanced by providing examples and illustrations, Barbara may trace the path the food travels by directing Tim's hand from his mouth to his stomach and then to his anus. She may also draw a picture to illustrate how the food's consistency changes as it passes through the mouth and into the stomach. She may explain that the body will absorb the food's vitamins and minerals into bones and blood so that Tim will grow taller and stronger.

She may further explain that the bacteria in the intestines will change the food that the body doesn't need into a brown, soft, different-smelling substance called "feces" or "bowel movement." It's the bacteria that causes the feces to smell. It's the bacteria that carries the germs that may be transferred from the hands or fingernails into the mouth and can cause people to get sick with cramps or diarrhea. With no horrified outburst from Mom or Dad, Tim's childhood memories of potty training will not be fraught with guilt and shame.

Just as a side note: If Tim had been Tina, it would have been particularly important to explain that while urine is nearly germ-free, the bacteria of a bowel movement can cause an infection if it is introduced into the vagina. Wiping oneself from the front to the back is a good habit to reinforce.

Who would have thought that toilet training, an event that one hardly remembers, is such a significant benchmark for the way in which adults express their sexuality? Yet the results of a person's childhood toilet training experience are clearly evidenced in the way that they take pride in their appearance and in their attitude about caring for their body. Toilet training also sets the scene for learning to follow instructions in a healthy, orderly fashion. But what's most important is that this is *the first time that a child assumes complete control of his or her body.*

The muscles and nerves that control the child's voluntary elimination may not be developed until about two or three years of age. Physically, some children may be ready, but they will *choose not to be responsive* because of or in spite of a parent's plea or demand. Children *choose* whether to let go or hold back. They *choose* whether it's in their best interest to please an authority figure. Later in life they will make the same kind of choices in the way they express their sexuality.

For many parents, toilet training becomes a proclamation of their child's mastery. It may become a source of stress for parents who encounter resistance from the child. As the following Golden Opportunity illustrates, relaxed parents allow their children to signal the appropriate time for potty training.

✳ ✳ ✳Despite his parents' coaxing, three-year-old Joel has no interest in the potty. In fact, the potty has become a place to store special possessions. It also is a throne for his favorite Teddy who, says Joel, has no desire to be potty trained. One day Dad forgets to lock the bathroom door while he is on the toilet and Joel roams into this forbidden scenario. Joel stares at Dad as though he has discovered a great buried treasure. Dad is flustered and uncomfortable. Dad's secret is out: He is human. He actually defecates like the rest of the world. "What are you doing?" Joel asks. Still startled by the intrusion, Dad responds cryptically, "I'm moving my bowels!" "Where are you moving them?" Joel asks. "Well," Dad says as he attempts to cover his exposed body with a newspaper, "I'm not actually moving them, I'm really making a bowel movement in the toilet." "Can I see?" asks Joel. "No," snaps Dad. "Please, Dad, please, can't I see? Is it bad?" "No, Joel it's not bad but I'm . . ." Dad searches for a word, "embarrassed because it's private. Bowel movements are what big people do into the toilet. It looks just like the bowel movement you make in your diaper."

Joel pleads tearfully with Dad, "P-l-e-a-s-e, can't I see it?" Finally, Dad succumbs, scuffling with the toilet tissue and attempting to pull up his pants while still guarding his nudity with the newspaper. He squirms as Joel peers into the toilet. "Wow," exclaims Joel, "that's a big bowel movement!" "Yeah," responds Dad, like a defensive adolescent, and then retorts, "at least I don't do it in my diaper like you do." With that, Joel asks if he can go on the toilet just like Daddy. "Sure!" exclaims Dad. Happily surprised, Dad holds Joel on the seat while Joel makes his first official toilet deposit. There are squeals of joy. Dad is exuberant. He praises Joel repeatedly. "Don't let go," Joel warns, "I don't want to fall in." "You won't fall in," Daddy promises. "As soon as you are finished we will go to the store to buy you a seat that fits on top of this one that will be just the right size for you. Or you can use your potty if you want." "No," Joel declares, "the potty is for Teddy. It's not for real big people!"

While this Dad was not the ideal portrait of the relaxed parent, both he and his son learned many important lessons. Dad learned that:

- Parents are their children's best role model.
- Children learn best by example.
- Children take pride in imitating their parents.
- Children see no shame in their body and how it functions, unless taught otherwise.
- A child's understanding is literal (for example, "moving my bowel").
- Children can discover Golden Opportunities, too.

In the words of Eastern philosophy: "When the student is ready, a teacher appears."

A sensitive parent is aware of a child's readiness to assume a new skill. In the case of toilet training, children may notify a parent that their diaper needs to be changed or may ask when they can wear underpants just like their big brother or sister. One thing is certain: When children are ready, they will let you know. When a child is forced to do something by an authority figure who misguidedly withholds love and affection as a punishment for failure, an unhealthy cycle in achieving love is established. When children are forced to perform beyond their ability, a power conflict is created.

Freud refers to the toilet training period, when children are more concerned about elimination than any other aspect of their life, as the anal stage. Just as an infant in the oral stage must be lovingly nourished by means of sucking in order to move forward in a healthy sequence, Freud believes that a relaxed attitude toward potty training will discourage the development of a rigid, negative, and often controlling personality in later life.

Recognizing their power to control parents, some children may request to sit on the potty and then climb down to leave a deposit on the bathroom floor. Some may defiantly refuse to submit to the pleas and bribes of their parents. Later in life, the manner in which the child controlled the dynamics of this event may directly affect the way in which he or she responds to the give-and-take of an intimate relationship. Early messages of holding back and letting go may become a precursor for an adult male who is so anxious to please that he may have difficulty achieving an erection or prolonging the release of ejaculation. An adult female who is still holding back and defying authority may be so in control that she is unable to permit herself to experience the joy of an orgasm.

I recently conducted a teacher's workshop during which I discussed the notion that early negative messages about toilet training may impair our willingness to release ourselves in the adult bedroom. After the session, a teacher handed me a folded note, hugged me, and left. Later that day I read the note: "For the first time in my life, I believe I understand my extremely controlled behavior in the bedroom. I have never been able to let go and be intensely intimate with my husband. I am the product of compulsive parents who, to this day, continue to recall my "defiant" attitude in holding out against their persuasion, whether it was walking, talking, or even toilet training. I came here today to learn about kids, but I wound up learning something about myself. I feel ready to rethink my sexual behavior. Thank you, again and again."

NUDITY: THE BARE FACTS

I'm in my office, listening to a high-intensity saga related to children's nudity. Ron and Tina left their two children, ages three and seven, in the care of Grandmother, who was visiting from up North. At noon, Tina receives a call at work to return home immediately. As she enters the house, she sees that Grandmother is in a rage. The children's faces are streaked with tears.

Grandmother summarizes the saga: "It's been beastly hot to-day. Your neighbor invited the children to play under her sprinkler. I dressed them in bathing suits and sent them off with a shirt, thongs, and a towel. Later, I went to check on them. There they were," she exclaims, *"your* son and *your* daughter and your neighbors' kids. One looks to be eleven or twelve years old. They were *all* running around the garden sprinkler *stark naked!*

"I insisted that the children put on their towels and come home. There was a lot of arguing and crying. I finally literally had to pull them from this nudist camp and wrap them in towels to bring them back home.

"God knows," Grandmother exclaims, "you weren't raised like this." "You're right," Tina replies. "I apologize, Mother, not for my children's comfort with their own bodies, but for not explaining to you in advance the rules that we accept in our home. Ron and I have developed new values. We think it's healthy for our children to enjoy their bodies without a feeling of shame, and to see how different bodies look, especially as they grow and change." Morals of saga:

- Before leaving your children to the charge of a surrogate parent, you should clearly explain your sexual values, from nudity to self-pleasuring to appropriate touch.
- Accept as a fact that new values may not be accepted by old teachers.
- Hold fast to what you believe is your truth.
- Children and parents can disagree on certain values and still love one another.
- It's important for your children to know that Mom and Dad agree on the same sexual values.
- Rescue your children from the hands of dissenters with loving affirmation: "While Grandmother loves and cares for you very much, we do not always agree on what is best for you. Daddy and I are happy that you can choose to play under the sprinkler, *with* or *without* your bathing suit. Grandmother didn't know our rules. Now she does. Next time there will be no problems." Mom hugs children. Children hug Mom. Mom hugs Grandmother. Grandmother now must decide how she will accept this new information.

How was nudity handled at your home? Did Mom and Dad dress behind closed doors? Did you ever shower with your mother or father? Were the genitals viewed as a mystery only to be touched or examined by a physician?

The messages you received as a child have helped form your belief system today. When a child is young, there is a lot to be learned from showering together. Some of the stories shared in our adult sexuality groups are hilarious. Deborah recounted an incident of showering with her three-year-old daughter Cindy. The child stroked the soft patch of pubic hair between Mom's legs and coquettishly mewed like the family's newborn kitten. This reasonable association became a Golden Opportunity. Deborah laughed and agreed that the pubic area does look and feel like a kitty's fur. Deborah then went on to explain that baby girls are born with no hair around their labia (lips of vagina) and baby boys have no hair around their penis, but that when they grow to be as big as Cousin Judy or Cousin Brett, some hair begins to grow in that area. When Cindy gets to be a grown woman, she, too, will have a soft patch of short, curly hair, just like Mommy. (Mom could add that this hair is called pubic hair because it only grows in the area that is called the pubic area.)

Deborah invited Cindy to touch the downy hair on Deborah's arms and legs as well as the new growth under her arms, reiterating that Cindy would develop and look like Mom when she got older. After the shower, Deborah reinforced the lesson with books that illustrated how boys develop into men and girls into women. Showering with parents is an ideal time for little children to see how adults look and to understand what to expect from their body as they mature.

I recommend bathing or showering with children only if you feel comfortable doing so. Children are perceptive, and they can easily discern the mixed messages of a forced situation. There are many mixed messages associated with sexuality, as it is. So, please, let your comfort level be your guide.

Edith, single mother of four-year-old Aaron, cringed at the thought of showering with her son, yet she thought it would be instructive for Aaron to see adults of both sexes undressed. The next time her brother Chuck and his family came for a weekend visit, Edith encouraged Chuck to share the bathroom and shower with Aaron. Edith's brother managed to direct the conversation to create a Golden Opportunity.

❋ ❋ ❋Uncle Chuck claims that he has forgotten his razor and asks Aaron if Aaron's mom might have one to spare. Aaron produces a razor and Chuck invites Aaron to help him shave. Chuck and Aaron playfully apply the shaving cream to one another's faces. Chuck asks if Aaron's mom uses the same kind of shaving cream. "Funny," Chuck says as he clowns in the mirror, "since your mom had this razor, I thought she needed to shave her beard every day, like we men do." Aaron roars with laughter. Chuck has set the stage for a boy-to-man talk. "Does Mom's face feel like this?" Chuck asks as he directs Aaron's hand across his prickly beard. "No!" Aaron responds with more laughter. "Women sure are different from men, aren't they?" "Yep!" Aaron responds.

Chuck continues, "We men grow hair on our face, arms, legs, and under our arms. Do you have any hair there yet?" Chuck checks out Aaron's body while Aaron giggles. "Nope, no hair yet, but you will have it when you get to be big like me and Cousin Perry and Uncle Kit." Chuck finishes his shave and uses his finger as a razor edge to remove the shaving cream from Aaron. Chuck turns on the shower and invites Aaron to join him. "We guys can use a good shower after a shave." Aaron and Chuck remove their shorts and shower together while Chuck continues his banter. "Hey, Aaron, you know where else we men grow hair! Yep, we men, like Uncle Allan, Cousin Dean, and I, have hair around our penis." More laughter. "Hey, Aaron, how's your penis doing?" Loud laughter. "Well, it looks pretty good to me. It looks just right for a four-year-old guy. When you get to be a big guy like me, your penis will get to look something like mine." Aaron looks at Chuck's penis without laughing. Finally, Aaron asks, "How come Mom doesn't have a penis? Did it fall off? Can my penis fall off, too?"

And so, a real concern was uncovered—a normal typical concern of a child of three or four or five. Perhaps that's why Aaron has been holding his penis so frequently. Perhaps that's why he's been so curious about playing doctor. Uncle Chuck did a superb job as Aaron's sexuality educator. He provided honest answers to honest concerns.

QUESTIONS OF MODESTY

Propriety means covering up or protecting parts of the body that are perceived to be sexually enticing. If we lived in Samoa, the rules for propriety would be to cover the navel. Our culture happens to require that the female breasts (especially the nipples), the penis, the vulva, and the buttocks be kept under wraps.

Usually, by the age of five, children recognize the accepted standards of propriety and develop their own sense of modesty. All at once they will demand to go to the bathroom alone. They may close the door to their room for privacy and will put their belongings in hiding places.

If, however, your child is a product of a sexually liberated household where bathroom sharing and nudity is nonchalantly accepted, you may find that you now have to initiate a few rules to restrain your child's uninhibited free spirit. I suggest that you explain to your children that while nudity is perfectly fine at home or when skinny-dipping at a lake, it's not OK to expose the parts of your body that are covered by your underwear at any other time. In fact, even though your underwear covers more of your body than a swimsuit, it's not OK to show your underwear to anyone but Mommy, Daddy, indicated significant other persons, and the doctor.

You may use a "What if" game of reasoning with your child to illustrate the point of propriety: "What if Daddy went to church without any clothes? What if you went to school without any clothes?"

The "what if" game helps children reason out what may happen in advance of an actual situation. Also, it allows a child to rehearse, in his or her mind, what to do and say when faced with the "What if" situation: "What if the gardener asked to see your penis?"

I recommend to my clients that they establish rules of propriety by the time their children are four years old and preferably earlier. It is about this time that a child identifies a penis with being male, and breasts and vulva with being female. Some children see their buttocks as a neutral part of the anatomy. It's a good idea to tell children that "flashing" or "mooning" to gain attention or to play a prank is not appropriate behavior. For those children who need some guidance, do so in a good-humored manner: "What if I were to flash my buttocks in front of all your friends at nursery school?" The "What if" game will help your child understand that clothes are not only worn for warmth and protection, but also to meet our cultural standards.

WHEN NUDITY IS UNHEALTHY

A teenage boy could feel great discomfort (even though he may not say it) when he sees his mother undressed. The same may hold true if a teenage girl views her naked father. I caution parents that the naturalness of nudity becomes unhealthy and a danger to a child when it is interpreted to be seductive and exploitative. Such behavior is not always easy to identify. Perhaps this glimpse into my office will better illustrate what I mean.

It's hard to believe that Terry, with her model-like figure, is the mother of 13-year-old Ginny, 11-year-old Keith, and 6-year-old Jon. Terry has brought Ginny to the center to obtain contraception. Behind closed doors, Ginny expresses anger that her mom even suspects that she is having intercourse. "Just because Mom thinks that everyone is after *her* body, doesn't mean that everyone else has sex on their mind!"

Ginny continues, "We're embarrassed to bring our friends to our house. You never know what Mom will be wearing—or *not* wearing: Brett's friends think Mom is a tease. When Brett complains, Mom laughs and says, 'If your friends think it's too hot to play in my kitchen, let them play elsewhere.' I know Scott feels funny when Mom cuddles up to him when he's watching TV. Dad says that Mom can't help it if she's beautiful and sexy. He thinks it's all a big joke."

Terry's seductive demeanor has passed the point of propriety. Adolescents who are struggling with their own sexuality may become confused and guilt-ridden when, upon viewing a parent's nudity, their hormones dictate a sexual surge. A child can become obsessed with these forbidden fantasies, which may become sexually debilitating later in life. As adults, these children may suppress their sexual desires for fear of acting inappropriately. They may also act aggressively to relieve their sexual frustrations.

Ginny's mother has been socialized to be seductive. She can recall wooing her parents, charming her teachers, enchanting her bosses, and captivating her husband. She has always felt comfortable about her body. At first, she rejects the notion that her behavior could be interpreted as exploitative and seductive. As we began to explore the ways in which she sexualizes her relationships, however, Terry decides to exercise greater discretion in certain circumstances. Everyone benefits from this situation where the children became the teachers.

I encourage parents who have struggled with questions of nudity to ask themselves:

- Do I feel comfortable?
- Does my child appear to feel comfortable?
- Do I feel it is appropriate?
- Would I have wanted my parents to provide this opportunity?

If the answer to these questions is "Yes," then continue to follow your inclination. But if you answer "Yes" to the following questions, I strongly suggest that you rethink your values.

- Is my behavior a way of affirming my sexuality?
- Is my behavior a way of acting out sexual feelings such as frustration, inadequacy, loneliness, or anger?
- Is my behavior a way of acting out sexual needs, like the need to be touched, appreciated, or admired?

- Does my child appear titillated, embarrassed, or otherwise uncomfortable?
- Does my child appear overly curious?
- Does my child avert his or her eyes from me?
- Does my child make covert comments like, "Aren't you cold?" or overt comments like, "Shouldn't you cover up?"

SEX PLAY: IS THERE A DOCTOR IN THE HOUSE?

Playing doctor is one of those thorny issues that continues to perplex parents. And why not? I bet playing doctor outranks "Monopoly" in popularity and universal appeal. One parent in our sexuality group shared with us a "playing doctor" story involving her five-year-old son Andrew. Mom had been suspicious of Andrew's activities behind closed doors. She kept insisting that he keep the door open when he and his friends played in his room, but Andy kept "forgetting" to honor the request.

One day, when her three- and five-year-old nieces joined Andrew and his friends behind closed doors, Mom became alarmed. Each time she would open the door, it would mysteriously close again. Finally, Mom's anxiety could no longer be contained. She put her ear to the closed door and distinctly heard Andy say, "OK, Ms. Jones, we are now going to take your temperature."

Mom's heart was pounding. In an instant she thought of all the things she *should* do and *could* do.

- Should she rush in and rescue "Ms. Jones" and punish Andy?
- Should she knock on the door and give them warning that she's coming in?
- Should she not enter, but ask through the door, "What are you doing?"
- She could open the door and, in a controlled and calm manner, ask everyone to go home.
- She could ask whose idea this was and see that the child is punished.

- She could spank Andy in front of his friends to teach them all a lesson.
- She could express her surprise and disappointment, using shame and guilt as a deterrent for continuing this play.
- She could turn this experience into a Golden Opportunity.

Mom had rehearsed her response to an event of this kind and she was prepared to create a Golden Opportunity.

✳ ✳ ✳Mom knocked on the door and announced that she was entering the room. When she stepped inside, she saw that her three-year-old niece (alias Ms. Jones) was naked from the waist down, as was one of Andrew's friends. Mom looked at Andy and calmly said, "Dr. Andrew Stone, you are needed in surgery. Will you please come with me." Turning to the other children, Mom said, "You patients can get dressed now. The doctor has been called away for an emergency." Mom guided the frightened doctor into the next room. Smiling, she said, "Don't look so frightened. I'm not angry, and you are not in trouble." Andy now looked both relieved and puzzled. "I understand that you are only playing a game, but I'm concerned that your friend's mother and your cousin's mother may not want their children to play this game. In fact, *I'd prefer that you not play this game, either.* If you would like to play doctor, I'll be glad to be the nurse while you examine our baby or Aunt Sue's baby or even Mrs. Taylor's new baby. But, for now, I'd like you and your friends either to model with the clay or play kickball."

Please note that Andy's Mom immediately defused Andy's anxiety by *accepting,* but not *approving,* his activity. Mom said that she'd *prefer* that Andrew not play this game. In the future, Andy may *choose* to play doctor again, although he knows Mom would prefer that he does not. She also has given him the option to play doctor with her guidance and assistance as his "nurse," which would provide further Golden Opportunities.

Some sexologists believe that sex-play is a healthy experience for children and should not be discouraged if these rules of play are instituted:

- Sex-play should never be forced upon another.
- Sex-play should be initiated only if it is desired by both (or all) the children.
- Objects should not be inserted into any orifice.
- The play must be stopped if a child becomes aggressive or abusive. (These rules of sex-play are as imperative for adults as they are for children.)

Other "sexperts" believe that sex-play should not be encouraged and that other options for sex exploration should be offered (for example, examining a baby with mother's supervision). No research exists to prove or disprove the virtues or ills of children playing such games. There is, however, data compiled from thousands of interviews that reveal that the greatest danger is *the manner in which a parent addresses the situation.* Children who have been severely punished, ridiculed, and embarrassed clearly recall, as adults, their guilt, shame, and confusion. It's just the kind of message from childhood that negatively colors an adult perspective of sexuality.

One more note: Mom assigned Andrew the responsibility of taking control of the situation. Andrew's dignity was kept intact as he returned to the room and offered two options for alternative play. One option would allow the children to play out the feeling through the medium of clay. The other option would allow the children to release their anxiety and desire for body contact through the physical activity of kickball.

When Mom and Andy returned to the room, Mom told the children that she understood how interesting it is to play doctor. "When I was a little girl, I played doctor, too. I wanted to know, just as you do, how boys and girls look different from one another when they are undressed. But it's not a good idea to poke inside each other because someone can get hurt. And some mommies and daddies won't like the idea of your getting undressed to play this game. So, Andrew has two good ideas for other games you can play now." The discussion was ended and the children moved on to the next activity.

A question now arises. Should Mom inform all the children's parents about what has occurred? If I were the parent, I would want to know for a variety of reasons. I would have appreciated learning how Andy's mom handled the situation. The incident also would be my signal to initiate a matter-of-fact discussion about the body and its changes. I would be motivated to buy books with photos of bodies at different ages and stages. And I would either purchase or create, with my child's assistance, a soft, stuffed, gender-specific doll. A note of caution: There are some parents who may be blaming and disapproving of your actions. In turn, they may forbid their children play at your home again. Personally, I'd prefer to lose such a parent as an acquaintance. And while I would feel badly about the consequences the child may reap, there is always the chance that my behavior may act as a role model for the parent to rethink his or her values. You must weigh the risks and the benefits. There is always the possibility that the parent will opt for something like the following Golden Opportunity.

✳ ✳ ✳ Five-year-old J.P. has been discovered playing doctor. Mom and Dad buy J.P. anatomically correct dolls, along with a child-size green surgical scrub suit and a doctor's kit. Dad and Mom undress the dolls with J.P. and identify all of the body parts. The dolls have breasts and nipples, underarm and pubic hair, as well as a vagina, penis, and anus. Many of the dolls come equipped with sanitary pads for the girls and interchangeable penises (circumcised and uncircumcised), along with a rolled condom in the back pocket for the boys. Dad and Mom also have purchased a doctor's kit with a stethoscope, which actually can transmit the heart sounds to the ears. They listen to one another's heartbeats, take each other's pulse, and teach J.P. how to read a thermometer. Rules of safety, hygiene, and first aid are discussed. They include some "What if" activities like "What if you cut your finger?" "What if you put this thermometer into the anus of one of these dolls?" "What if this penis is not circumcised?"

Can you recall your confusion when you were caught innocently engaging in some "naughty" activity, not understanding what you had done to elicit such attention and reprimand? Children who explore one another should not be punished. This is no more a sexual assault than the wonderment displayed when a child tries to fly like a bird or disassembles a radio to see how it works.

Non-sexual curiosity about the way the body works is usually first evidenced when the child is about two-and-a-half years old and begins to explore himself. At age six or seven, it is evidenced again when children explore each other. While it is more common for children of the same sex rather than of the opposite sex to examine one another, this stage is usually short-lived. After the age of seven, children usually develop a strong sense of modesty and privacy. At adolescence the curiosity is again reawakened, but this play is more sexual in nature.

Parents who casually supervise their young children at play can gently guide them so that they do not become frightened or over-whelmed. A parent can step in and suggest, for example, "I think the doctor is pushing too hard on the patient's stomach. The mommy knows how hard to push so that the baby can come out of the vagina." If you are surprised by a discovery of sex-play, isolate the activity, as Andrew's mother did, and respond as you would if you had discovered your child innocently dismantling the telephone. Relax. Make this moment a Golden Opportunity for learning to-gether. Perhaps years later your child's unbridled curiosity will be rewarded as he or she graduates from medical school.

FANTASY AND PRETENDING: THE WORLD OF MAKE-BELIEVE

Curiosity, pretending, and fantasy are stimulated at an early age. A child who is encouraged through play to appreciate sensuous plea-sure will mature into an adult with a heightened capacity for sexual arousal. We have already talked about the merits of mirror games to affirm a child's sense of identity. In addition, there are the "close your eyes and guess" games, in which a child is asked to identify:

- The sounds of nature, music, animals, humanity
- The tastes of foods of different flavors and consistency and temperatures

- The feel of velvet, silk, cotton, feathers, sandpaper, rope
- The play of finger paints, clay, sand, water
- The aroma of perfume, salt air, flowers, pine needles

The blending of sensuous sensitivity with the ability to fantasize increases both the physical and spiritual pleasures of adult lovemaking.

I always suggest to clients that they include fantasy and playfulness in their lovemaking. "Revive the curious child that is hibernating within," I tell them. "I don't know how to fantasize," they say, "and if I did, I'd probably feel too guilty to share this with my lover." I then ask if they have ever daydreamed. "Of course," they will respond. The wholesome act of daydreaming is the forerunner to fantasy. And fantasy is the precursor to playfulness.

To help clients release their natural impulse to fantasize, I ask them to create an ambiance designed to recapture the natural sensory responses of their childhood. I often suggest that they immerse their body in a warm, scented bath, dry their body with a velvety towel, and lovingly apply body oils from the face to the toes. Next I suggest mellow music, an aromatic candle or incense, and a leisurely body massage.

Somewhere along the way we lose touch with the sensuous pleasures that trigger sexual responsiveness. Sensual responsiveness frees a person to daydream . . . to fantasize . . . to be playful . . . to enjoy their God-given sexual potential.

Curiosity, imagination, and playing "make-believe" provide a child with a healthy channel to act out thoughts and feelings. Play is serious business for children. A child's ability to pretend and fantasize is encouraged when a parent provides the stimulation of soft dolls, building blocks, puppets, stuffed animals, and assorted objects such as plastic dishes, child-safe tools, and cast-off adult clothes in which to dress.

Through play, children explore the male and female qualities of their personality and actually *rehearse adult behavior* for the future. Listening to children play can give parents a pretty good idea of how they are responding to the pushes and pulls of life. The three-year-old girl who is obsessed with self-pleasuring scolds her dolly for touching her "gina." The four-year-old boy who can't measure up to his father's expectations reprimands his playmate for acting like a wimp. The five-year-old child who fears his or her sexual attraction to the parent of the opposite sex fashions a cave from a carton in which she or he alone can hide. The six-year-old bedwetter kicks the stuffed dog for refusing to become housebroken. The seven-year-old whose parents are in custody battle creates puppet characters who argue, curse, and belittle one another.

The child who tearfully describes a monster hiding under the bed may really want a hug from Mom and Dad or just reassurance that both parents are home. The child who claims that the dog urinated in her bed would like dry, clean sheets, but also doesn't want to be punished for the bedwetting accident.

To this day, there is a "food ghost" who continues to reside in our household. It strikes during the night when I am sleeping and devours an assortment of delectable treats. Occasionally, he leaves a note on the refrigerator door stating that the food ghost strikes again. He signs the note with a smudged fingerprint. The elusive ghost has outfoxed our calorie-conscious family for years.

Lily, a mother in our sexuality group, tells of her life-enhancing experience through fantasy. "I grew up as an only child surrounded by many teachers and kindly authority figures. My mother recalls that at the age of two I created my imaginary friend DoeDi. I looked to DoeDi for advice and frequently attributed my misbehavior to her.

"We have pictures of me scolding this imaginary person for wetting her diaper. Mom would ask me to remind DoeDi that big girls don't have accidents. Mom remembers me responding that DoeDi didn't want to be a big girl. Mom knew from that response that she had better not push the toilet training process until I was ready to assume my role as a big girl.

"DoeDi comforted me when I was frightened and played with me when I was lonely. The whole family mourned the passing of DoeDi when she mysteriously disappeared on my sixth birthday. At age six, I didn't have time for DoeDi because I was so preoccupied with making human friends.

"Sometimes I still playfully call on DoeDi's assistance when

I'm in search of a parking space, or when I'm challenged beyond my abilities."

The only time daydreaming or fantasy is a concern is when it becomes an obsession and is used as a form of isolation. Seven-year-old Ilene is painfully shy. Rather than risk playing with other children, she wanders away and busies herself in thought. Often in class she emotionally removes herself from student projects by staring off into space as though she is daydreaming. In order to encourage Ilene to partake in interpersonal activities, Ilene's parents built her, from a cardboard carton, a puppet theater and created handcrafted puppets through which Ilene could express herself. The puppets became a safe and playful communicator of Ilene's inner concerns. The puppets disclosed her fear of failure at school. In class, the teacher encouraged Ilene to use the hand puppets to deliver oral reports. Ilene forgot her inhibitions as she became the voice for the inanimate characters. Her teacher and classmates applauded Ilene's skill in maneuvering the puppets. Their appreciation elevated Ilene's confidence and self-esteem. In a few months, Ilene was able to participate in class without the aid of her puppet friends.

Fantasies provide opportunities to savor an experience without physically acting it out. These thoughts are safe expressions. No matter how absurd, bizarre, or disturbing they may be, there is normal compulsion to act upon them. It's important to remember that *all thoughts are normal* and are not expressions of uncontrollable urges that must become realities. In fact, *fantasy may provide a safeguard against a compulsion to act inappropriately in real life.*

Later in life, fantasy adds magic to a relationship. You may find it a safe way to express desires upon which you will never act. Or, you may find them to be a joyful expression upon which you can expand and enrich the pleasures of adult lovemaking. Fantasy can be a priceless aphrodisiac.

Parents often ask, "How can I motivate my children to pretend?" There are many opportunities. As a young child, did you ever dress in disguises or in adults' clothing? Did you ever watch your Mom and Dad mow the lawn or lift weights and later imitate their feats of accomplishment behind closed doors?

It is said that imitation is the greatest form of flattery. By the age of two, children love to mimic their parents' actions. You can turn this natural inclination into dozens of Golden Opportunities, such as those that follow:

✳ ✳ ✳Create a treasury of resources that will titillate a child's imagination by providing a wardrobe of old clothes, discarded jewelry, and, of course, a full-length mirror. Children especially love hats of all kinds, from helmets to flowing millinery creations. Set aside a "let's pretend" area in the attic, basement, or playroom. Tools, instruments, and cleaning utensils scaled to size and child-safe are but a few accessories that can enhance the fantasy. Additional amenities may include a Polaroid camera, an audio-cassette recorder or a video recorder to preserve the magic of disguise.

There are endless opportunities for parents of children to share in the pretending activities. An alert ear and eye will open the doors and windows to your child's thoughts and feelings.

MOMMA'S BOY AND DADDY'S GIRL: SEXUAL IDENTITY AND FANTASY

Make-believe is a healthy opportunity for a child to explore and confirm his or her gender identity. Sexually healthy children are encouraged to experience all levels of their maleness and femaleness so that they can tap any of these qualities to suit the occasion.

The term *androgeny* is used to describe a person who displays traditional male *and* female characteristics. Androgenous individuals respond with equal grace to the role of the initiator or the nurturer, the aggressor or the pacifist. This ideal, integrated state of being can be fostered by the example you set for your children (that is, it's OK for Dad to cry and it's OK for Mom to adjust a carburetor). It can also be established by providing children with opportunities to pretend.

Boys and girls love to assume a different identity. Even as an adult, it is great fun to masquerade for an evening. "But," asks a mother from the sexuality group, "how can I convince my husband that it's OK for our five-year-old son to go to a Halloween party dressed in my clothes?" I suggest that she explain to her husband the virtues of "make-believe," and that if he is still concerned that his son has a conflicted sexual identity, she should assure him that studies prove that it is far too early to make such an assumption based on such evidence.

Here again we may look to Freud for advice. Perhaps your child is creatively resolving his natural Oedipal urge to steal Mom from Dad. He cannot be his mother's lover, so he's going to step into her shoes to see how they fit on this appropriate occasion for disguise, Halloween. When he sees how unfit he is for the role, he will align himself with Dad and begin to emulate his father's behavior. I tell her to be glad that at five years of age your son has a definite awareness of what is male and female. Far from being a cause for Dad's alarm, perhaps the child's choice of costume is a way of confirming his masculinity.

Both sexes have a natural and *harmless* curiosity about the costume of the opposite sex. You might say that the child is trying on the moccasins of the Indian to get a sense of another's identity. Disguised in the clothes of another character, the child is developing another point of view, allowing him to experience another's feelings, thoughts, fears, and joys. This awareness of others will expand in adulthood into the ability to empathize, to feel compassion, to be considerate, nurturing, and finally to feel love for another. Worry not; your child will not be locked into his fantasy identity any more than you and I were entrapped as children when we dressed as a dragon or an angel for Halloween. *Pretending promotes thoughtfulness and sensitivity unlike any other activity.*

By the time your son is six and soon to be seven, he should have more clearly defined his sexual identity. On the other hand, if he repeatedly and surreptitiously continues to wear Mom's makeup, jewelry, or high-heeled shoes, if he always chooses the mother role in games with other children, and if he avoids playing with same-sex friends, he may be experiencing a sexual identity problem. As a first step, a male figure should spend more time with him in traditional man-boy activities, such as bowling, bicycling, and exercising. He should be encouraged and praised for each activity he attempts.

For the single mother who cannot identify a significant male model in her family, I suggest Big Brother as an organization that can provide the surrogate masculine image that this child may be seeking.

Also seek school settings where the teacher is male; find a baby-sitter who is male, if you can, or one who has brothers who might interact with your son. For the single father with the same concern for his daughter, there is Big Sister, offering the same service.

This is not a time to panic. This is a Golden Opportunity to assist your child in clarifying his gender identity. If you were to ask your son why he chooses this behavior, he may naïvely explain that it's more fun to dress as a mommy because mommies wear prettier clothes than daddies and they are allowed to put on lipstick and paint their face. At this point, the parent can agree that mommies do have prettier clothes and jewelry, but that daddies aren't supposed to dress like mommies. Use the "What if" technique of reasoning: "What if Daddy went to work dressed like a mommy? What would people say? What would they think of Daddy?" An older child may have the same notion. He may even wish he could be a woman. Many children believe that they can switch their gender by imitating the dress code of the opposite sex.

Once children understand that their gender is permanent and that they will always be male or female despite the clothes that they wear, they begin to style their behavior after the parent of the same sex.

An older child will benefit from a discussion of gender-appropriate behavior. It can begin with "It's really neat to be a boy. What kinds of things do boys do that most girls don't do? What do you most like doing as a boy?" Despite the limitations imposed upon people by sexual stereotyping, this would be an appropriate time for you to identify male behavior as illustrated in books and magazines. The most important issue here is to help your child resolve his confusion in a loving, supportive manner. Criticism and name-calling may sentence this child to a lifetime of sexual conflicts.

Says Sonia, the mother of seven-year-old Gregory, "My husband constantly teases Gregory with remarks like, 'Don't be such a sissy. Why don't you play football with the other boys?' He's always calling our son a wimp or a fag because he shows no interest in sports. He doesn't see anything wrong with our daughter acting like a tomboy, but every time I try to point out this contradiction, he either ignores me or claims that it's my fault that Gregory is a Momma's boy."

Isn't it interesting that today's society generally accepts tomboy behavior in a young girl, but labels a boy as a sissy if he does not live up to the sex role that society has dictated? Why is "Daddy's little girl" an expression of admiration, while "Mommy's boy" expresses ridicule? The sadness is the loss of human potential. Studies confirm that girls who are permitted to be tomboys in their youth usually grow up to be successful, balanced adults capable of taking greater risks, enjoying challenges, and embracing broader opportunities. History records many men who achieved monumental success that they have attributed to the love-security bond they shared with their mother. Franklin Delano Roosevelt, as well as Sigmund Freud, may be classified as Momma's boys, since they admittedly were their mother's favorite child.

The important thing is for a child to develop naturally to be the best that she or he is capable of being. If not football, perhaps his preference is art, computers, music, or water sports. If not dolls, perhaps her preference is brain surgery or law. If you're concerned that encouraging girls to play with trucks and boys with dolls is going to lead them down the path of homosexuality, relax. Exploring *all* their interests will allow them to become fully functioning human beings. It will also give them insights into how and why the opposite sex responds as it does.

Forcing children to engage in gender-specific activities only confuses them as they seek to establish their sexual identity. It may have precisely the *opposite effect* of what parents intended. These children are often discouraged from expressing their full range of emotions and are told, "What are you afraid of? Don't act like a sissy," or "Don't yell, it's not ladylike." The excessive fear of homosexuality, known as homophobia, inhibits many parents: Dad never hugs son, and Mom is cautiously demonstrative. As adults, these children often question their natural inclination to be affectionate. They may remove themselves from intimate relationships, feeling unlovable or unworthy. Or they may become sexually aggressive or promiscuous, releasing their childhood anger at being rejected.

I recommended that Sonia and her husband, Karl, visit me for private counseling. "He'll never come," she insisted. "Well, simply tell him that I have a cure for sissy kids," I said. The next evening

Karl and Sonia came to my office. Karl set the stage: "I'm only here because I heard that you have a cure for Gregory." "How would you describe Gregory?" I asked. Karl thought for a moment. "He's a bright kid. He gives us no trouble except that he's a fag." "What do you mean when you say he's a fag?" I asked. "He's a wimp. He can't throw a ball; he has no interest in sports." "How did he get this way?" I asked. "Sonia's too soft with him," Karl said. "She should stop coming to his rescue. Gregory usually cries when I tell him to be a man. Sonia then hugs him and tells him it's OK. And so he thinks it's OK to be a sissy." "What kind of things do real men do?" I pursue. "What kind of things do *you* do, Karl?" "I'm in construction," he says. "I guess you can see that by just looking at me." Karl straightens his posture and flexes his muscles. "I bet Gregory thinks you're really strong," I continue. "I have a friend who's a world-renowned chef who just won a silver cup for weight-lifting," I comment. "Do you know that some football idols do hand embroidery, called needlepoint, for relaxation?" In fact," I continue, I heard that there are a lot of homosexuals in football. When those guys slap one another on the rear end it looks pretty gay to me. And when those linebackers look into the camera and say 'I love you, Mom' I can't help but think that they are Momma's boys." Karl laughs and shrugs.

"Karl," I continue quite seriously, "I'm afraid that you will push Gregory into a homosexual life-style unless you change your attitude toward him. Gregory is going through an important stage of his growth," I explain. "It's at this time in his life that he will make a decision about his sexual identity—a decision that may hold true for his entire life. When Gregory looks at you he sees a handsome, strong male figure who either can help him feel comfortable with his maleness or push him into a female frame of reference. Every time you call Gregory a wimp or a sissy or a fag, you are imprinting a promise in his brain. The promise is: When your father, whom you love and admire, tells you that you are a wimp, then you will, of course, obey his command. You are the wisest man in Gregory's life, Karl. Whatever you say, he believes it is correct. If he can't live up to your expectations, if you reinforce the fact that he is a fag, and if you force him to seek consolation for his failings from his only source of love—his mother—then he will fulfill your prophesy. He will do his best to obey you and that is to be a sissy."

I place my hands on top of Karl's and say, "I told you that I have a cure. I lied. Gregory is not sick. He is normal. I lied because I wanted to be able to look in your eyes and assure you that Gregory, like millions of other boys, is searching for his own identity. You couldn't have stepped forward at a better time to help Gregory find his way, because at seven years of age, now more than ever, Gregory is looking to you as his role model, his idol. I strongly recommend that you cool it on the sports and pursue together other manly interests, which can range from fishing to woodworking. This is a good time for Gregory to join the Boy Scouts and pursue a wide variety of activities, from music to camping. Gregory desperately needs your affirmation and affection. Your compliments will make him feel like a man. Your arm around his shoulder will make him feel like a worthwhile person. A hug from you will make him feel like a giant."

Karl is calm now. "Karl," I continue, "please do not ever call Gregory a sissy again. I can relate too many sad stories of children who could not bear up under the strain of name-calling. I know too many parents who wish they had another chance to tell their children of their love. Recently, a seven-year-old child ended his life because he could not cope with taunts about being overweight."

Karl wiped a tear from the corner of his eye. "Karl, you can help Gregory be the best Gregory he's capable of being. This is your Golden Opportunity to be the real man you really are." As Karl and Sonia leave, I ask Karl if I might give him a hug, and he awkwardly consents. "Hmmm," I say, "you're a good hugger. Gregory is a very lucky boy."

✳6✳

Leaving the Age of Innocence

Ellen, mother of 11-year-old Cynthia, had been waiting anxiously in the hall for 20 minutes when I arrived to open the office at 9 A.M. As it happened, my morning was free. We sipped coffee and listened to a relaxing musical tape as Ellen related her Friday night experience.

Ellen and her husband, Jay, encouraged sleep-over dates and slumber parties to provide daughter Cynthia, an only child, with an opportunity to see how others lived and to share with her contemporaries on an intimate level.

During the slumber party Cynthia had hosted the previous night, Ellen had had a premonition that events were taking an unusual turn. Melinda, the most physically and emotionally precocious of Cynthia's friends (she had been wearing a training bra for nearly a year) announced that she had just gotten her first period. Jody, an undeveloped 12-year-old with the sophistication of a young adult, had fallen madly in love with Mark, a 15-year-old "hunk" whom she had eyeballed at the bus stop. Nancy's older sister had just become engaged. And Cynthia had become fascinated with the thin patches of hair that were beginning to flower under her arms and around her vulva.

Acting on a whim, Ellen surreptitiously listened through the intercom in Cynthia's room just in case there was something that she should know that the girls were too self-conscious to reveal.

By 10:30 P.M., the girls had been locked in Cynthia's room for three hours. Between munching popcorn and wolfing down boxes of chocolate sandwich cookies. Between "gross me out" and "you are really weird," Nancy revealed a family secret. Her older sister had

76

become engaged because she was pregnant. "Why did she do that?" Cynthia naïvely asked. "I mean anyone can do IT, but that doesn't mean that you have to have a baby. I heard that you can just do it for fun." "It's supposed to be very relaxing, too," another added. "I heard it makes your zits go away."

"How do you think people do IT?" Cynthia asked. Nancy responded with a surprisingly good description of intercourse and explained that this opening (vagina), where a boy puts his "thing" to have sex, is the very place where Melinda's period was coming from. In order to understand where this special place is, she suggested they look at one another's vaginas. Melinda showed them her menstrual pad. After they commented with "yucks" and "gross," they asked her endless questions: "Does it hurt?" "When will you stop bleeding?" "What do you do with the bloody pads?" "Are you going to use those cigarette things instead of pads?"

"They then smuggled a box of Tampax into their room from my bathroom, and Melinda demonstrated how to put in a tampon," Ellen continued. "Melinda explained that inserting it was like "fucking," at which they all howled with laughter. "Maybe that's how your sister got pregnant," they exclaimed. Jody then called classmate Mark's house, intending to make a prank call, but hung up when his mother answered. Jody confessed to having dreamt about kissing Mark. "I put my tongue deep into his mouth and I thought I'd choke to death." They each then chose one of Cynthia's stuffed animals to help them demonstrate the art of kissing. "People can fuck animals," Jody said. "I read in the Bible that in the olden days some guys fucked sheep." "Gross me out!" they squealed. "Which do you think is worse," Jody asked, "fucking a sheep or sucking a dick?" "Oh, give me a break," they exclaimed in disgust. "Don't be such nerds," Jody added. "Everyone sucks dicks. Even your mother." "Oh, no! I don't believe it!" Cynthia said. "Wanna bet?" said Jody.

"As if this weren't enough," Ellen continued, "Jody told them about swallowing a man's ejaculate. She told them that it was called 'cum' and that every time a person sings 'Oh come, all ye faithful,' they really mean 'cum in my mouth.' Then they sang every song they could remember that had the word 'come' in the verse. When the hysteria died down, they called Mark's house again and were going to ask him if he ever dreamt of Jody and if he did, did it make him come in his sleep. Luckily, his mother answered again and told them that Mark was out for the evening.

"Then one of the girls produced an X-rated magazine she had borrowed from her brothers' room. They asked Melinda to compare her breasts with those featured in the photos. They each tried on Melinda's bra and asked to feel her breasts."

It was at this time that Ellen decided to make her presence known. By the time she had mustered her composure and entered the "den of iniquity," Cynthia had already shaved one of her legs. "The first thing I did to settle my nerves was some self-talk," Ellen told me. "I said to myself, 'Now, don't lose it. This is no different than the time you found Cynthia playing doctor seven years ago. They are only playing and exploring their changing sexuality. Nobody has been hurt. It's basically healthy fun.' When I felt calm, I knocked on the door and waited until they acknowledged my request to enter. I wanted them to know that I had an idea of what was happening, but I didn't want them to be embarrassed. I certainly didn't want them to know that I had been snooping. I smiled and walked directly to the intercom in Cynthia's room, feigning a gesture to adjust its dial. "One of you accidentally opened the speaker on the intercom," I said. The girls' eyes darted from one to the other. Finally, a single giggle erupted, which was followed by an explosion of nervous laughter. I told the girls that I hadn't heard much through the intercom, but that what I did hear sounded like the kind of questions I had had when I was their age. I told them that it was too late to talk about it now but that I would get them some books on the subject and we could talk about it later. As I exited and turned out the lights, encouraging them to go to sleep, I could hear their muffled laughter.

"It was a nightmare," Ellen said. "I don't know what time they finally fell asleep, but I dozed off at about 2 A.M."

"How can I help?" I asked.

"I need advice, I need information, and I need help," Ellen replied. "I need to be a biology teacher, sex educator, loving parent, and realistic mother. I'd most like to start a parent group," she suggested. "I'd feel so much more secure if I knew the right thing to say at the right time."

And so, Ellen became the initiator of our first parent group eight years ago. We have Cynthia and her friends to thank.

The group's mission was clear: "In order to safeguard a child's health and welfare, parents must assume their roles as their child's sexuality educators. All the parents expressed disappointment in not having taken a more active role earlier in their children's lives. They were sad and angry that they hadn't been better prepared by their own families. Once they forgave their parents, who were also victims of a sexually silent society, they were encouraged to learn that it's never too late to begin. They were enthused to realize that their sexuality education would not only help their children, but also would improve their own sexual relationships.

They used baby photographs of themselves as a way to connect with the past and their sexual history. One common myth that emerged was the Freudian notion that children were asexual from about age 7 through 12. These parents felt that there was no need to think about educating their children during this so-called latent period—until they heard about the conversation at Cynthia's slumber party. Whether it is due to improved nutrition, genetics, or a combination of both, coupled with a changing society and the sexualization of the media, children are biologically and emotionally maturing at an earlier age today than they did only a generation ago.

Luckily, Ellen became enlighted at a stage in Cynthia's life when Cynthia was eager for her parents' guidance and was willing to reveal her personal concerns. In a year or two, Cynthia probably will become more secretive and dependent on learning from her peers, as well as by trial and error. Now, however, Cynthia is willing to reveal to her mother her worries about scholastic achievement, her physical appearance, and the way she is treated by her friends. Cynthia, like most 11-year-olds, probably has unspoken fears of sexual abuse, divorce, and the death of a parent. Now she has an opening to disclose these fears.

The slumber party provided Ellen with a Golden Opportunity to help Cynthia handle the thorny issues of childhood: sex-play, self-touch, safe touch, nudity, street language, self-esteem, body image, curiosity, and exploration. All reappear in early adolescence and are combined with the influence of awakening sexual hormones.

BODY TALK: A GIRL AND HER ANATOMY

The first assignment presented to the parent group was that they share with their daughters factual information about the reproductive system. The challenge was to be creative and upbeat. The parents were cautioned that this assignment was particularly difficult because children are generally bored with laborious anatomy lessons and are far more interested in facts and feelings. I encouraged everyone to look for Golden Opportunities. A prize would be given for the most imaginative approach.

The following week, Samantha was declared the winner. She got a little help from a menstruating dog, but nonetheless she seized the occasion as a learning opportunity. Here is how Samantha's Golden Opportunity unfolded:

❋ ❋ ❋The family dog required menstrual hygiene products. Samantha applied the canine sanitary belt while Jennifer, her daughter, watched. "Aha," Samantha thought, "this is my Golden Opportunity." She started her conversation with an interesting fact: "Isn't it curious that all female animals are most at risk of becoming pregnant when they have their period, while human females are *least* at risk at that time of the month?" "How come?" her daughter asked. But when Samantha proceeded to explain, her daughter lost interest and said, "It really doesn't matter; let's talk about it later." "I probably made the explanation too complicated," Samantha admitted.

"Five days later, my daughter and I were having breakfast together," Samantha continued. "As Jennifer reached into the fruit bowl for some grapes, I pulled out a pear and declared, 'This is just what a uterus looks like.' 'That's nice,' my daughter replied, not terribly impressed. I put the pear on my abdomen and said, 'Isn't it amazing that a uterus this size can stretch to accommodate a full-size baby?' 'Yeah,' my daughter responded, somewhat more interested. 'You know,' I continued, 'you and I and every woman has a uterus about this exact size, located right inside the abdomen.' As my daughter continued eating the grapes, she placed a pear on top of her lower abdomen. Then I took two cherries and placed them on either side of her pear, enthusiastically explaining that the cherries could be the ovaries and the stems the fallopian tubes. Before you know it, my daughter and I had laughingly created the entire reproductive system using a celery stalk for the vagina and halves of a lemon for the breasts. We popped the pit out of the cherry and guided it along the fallopian tube and into the uterus. Since there was no sperm to be found, we conducted the pit through the celery and squeezed the cherry to add some juice and coloration to the 'menstrual flow.'

"It was such fun that we next took a banana and fashioned the male reproductive system from two prunes and two stems from the grapes. My daughter and I laughed until our sides hurt, and we learned a lot, too. Then I took out the schematic drawing of the female reproductive system (see the schematic drawing of female anatomy in the Appendix), and together we talked about all the parts and their function. Fruits and vegetables have taken on an entirely new dimension in our home," Samantha concluded with a chuckle.

THE RITES OF PASSAGE: GIRLS WILL BE WOMEN

The status of a female changes the moment she gets her first menstruation. Generally, between the ages of 11 and 13, at the onset of her first period (technically called *menarche*), a girl may be considered at risk for pregnancy. However, the notion that the onset of puberty constitutes reproductive ability is not true. Although there is no absolute yardstick by which to measure a pubescent's reproductive ability, a girl probably will not ovulate for a year or so after the onset of her first period.

When I conduct parent groups, I'm overwhelmed by the women's enthusiastic response to sharing memories about their first menstrual period. It is a touchstone that connects women of all ages. I ask:

- Where were you when it happened?
- Did you know what it was?
- What did you call it?
- Whom did you tell?
- What did you do?
- Were you wrongly advised that you would no longer be a virgin if you used tampons?
- Did you feel more feminine and mature, or did you feel less appealing and unclean?
- Was the event welcomed with a cheer and a rite of passage ceremony? Or, was it a source of embarrassment, confusion, and fear?

The time for a girl-to-woman talk is at pubescence, when a girl's breasts bud. On the vulva, straight hair appears, later to be followed by curly pubic hair. It's an awkward time for girls, who mature two years earlier than boys. Within a year of these first signs, the first menses should occur. With it come messages about being female that affect a woman's perspective of her femininety for the rest of her life. This is why a girl's preparation for this event is so important.

Some girls may feel more sensitive or tired during their period, while others feel energized and "sexy." Some can predict the onset of their period from body signs such as constipation, breast tenderness, and the appearance of a pimple or two, while others are caught unaware. It's a natural individualistic phenomenon that is distinctly female.

For generations, menstruation has been an unmentionable subject. Even today, two-thirds of American adults still believe that it is an inappropriate topic of conversation in mixed company, regardless of its context. One-quarter of those surveyed think it is improper to discuss anything associated with menstruation, *even within the family.*

I don't believe that any information about the body should be classified as unmentionable. Whenever I teach hygiene classes, I insist that boys as well as girls hear the same information at the same time. Sexually segregated classes only perpetuate the confusion, embarrassment and teasing that mar these wondrous events.

A relaxed discussion on menstruation provides Golden Opportunities to dispel myths and clarify cultural rites associated with becoming a menstruating woman. I have met women from homes in which the tradition was to slap a daughter across the face at the first onset of the menses. I've been told that this ancient custom is designed to return the blush of youth to the daughter's cheeks. Many of these young women who received no explanation, however, believed that they either were being punished for a mysterious misdeed or that the gesture confirmed menarche to be "the curse."

Other women, especially members of the Hebrew, Moslem, and Hindu sects, as well as the American Indians, continue to be told that they are "unclean" during their menses. These women are cautioned not to touch another person during those "dirty days" and are forbidden to engage in sexual activity during that time of the month. Observant Hebrew women are forbidden to have intercourse for a minimum of five days, which is calculated as a normal menstrual flow, plus seven days after to be certain that the flow has ceased. The woman is then required to submerge herself in a ritual bath (mikveh) before she can resume intimate bodily contact. Many women share with me their modern interpretation of the mikveh as a spiritual symbol to connote a nexus in their life. The nexus refers to the sadness in the completion of one cycle and the celebration, symbolized by the bath, of the beginning of a new cycle.

For generations, a menstruating woman was said to bring bad luck aboard a sailing vessel. She also was believed capable of sapping the strength from a man, dulling the blade of a sword, and destroying the blossom of a flower. Such unfounded "truths" depicting menstruating women as a danger to other people, objects, and even vegetation perpetuate negative feelings associated with the body and sexuality. Also implicit in these myths is the view that a woman's power to reproduce somehow diminishes a man's omnipotence. Menstrual blood reminds us all of the "magic" potential owned only by women. This perception of an imbalance of power is evidenced today in men who continue to diminish a woman's capabilities and status. I believe that the onset of menstruation is a cause for *celebration,* as is the emergence of *all* female powers!

It's fascinating for girls, as well as boys, to know that the monthly menstrual period will continue until a woman is 45 or 55 years old. It's also important that they understand that a woman will not be bleeding every day until that point, but only a few days a month, and that the real blood loss is minimal (no more than four to five tablespoons). A girl needs to know that her menstrual cycles will be irregular at first and that she will periodically miss a month or maybe more for the next year or two, until a 25- or 28-day cycle is established. Girls need to be reassured that they are not disabled during their menstruation.

For those who experience cramps before and during their period, I recommend moderate exercise and a balanced diet. There are herbal teas and nutritional supplements that reduce cramps and water retention, as well. As a general rule, I discourage prescription drugs, but do recommend antiprostaglandin medications for cramps when all else fails. In my work, I have found that girls often "inherit" a comfort level associated with menstruation. If they have been forewarned that it will be painful and debilitating, the prophecy will come true. If a girl has memories of her mother being confined to bed during those "cursed days," chances are that she will follow suit. Remember, children learn best by example.

Being attuned to the body's functions is important, however. I know one woman who is so aware of her body's rhythm that each month, 14 days before her period, she can feel a twinge in her lower abdomen (mittelschmerz or "middle pain") heralding the release of a mature egg into the fallopian tube at ovulation. She passed this information on to her daughter as a way of helping her daughter to know when her fertility was at its peak. While her daughter was not as aware of a twinge, she did experience a sense of pressure two weeks before the onset of her period each month. Her mom also taught her to check her cervical secretions at that time of the month. The clear, stretchy discharge, which occasionally held a tinge of blood, was another sign that ovulation had taken place. Rather than inculcating a foreboding of pain and discomfort, this mom and her daughter felt as though they were in synchrony with their body's signals. My guess is that the daughter's knowledge and awareness about menstruation, ovulation, and the body's rhythms will make her a much wiser user of contraceptives in the future.

TALKING ABOUT MENSTRUATION

No discussion about menstruation is complete without a demonstration of sanitary products. The products should be unwrapped, examined, and, if possible, applied over the clothes or to a doll. Tampons are frequently an issue of concern for parents. Some parents feel the insertion of a tampon is an invasion of their daughter's virginity. The fear is that the tampon will penetrate the thin membrane (hymen) at the entrance of the vagina that separates the vagina from the external genitals. The truth is that most hymens have an opening large enough to accommodate the insertion of a tampon. Hymens come in a variety of shapes, thicknesses, and sizes. Rarely does a hymen form an impenetrable barrier; if it did, the menstrual flow would not be able to exit from the uterus. Because the hymen stretches as a result of physical activity and self-pleasuring, it may have one opening or many openings. Therefore, the presence and condition of the hymen is not a true indicator of a woman's virginity.

My suggestion is that you weigh the pros and cons of tampons for your daughter. They are convenient and comfortable. They allow girls to partake of all activities, including swimming. In addition, inserting a tampon provides a health-related opportunity for girls to touch themselves. As explained in the chapter on comfort and self-touch, this becomes an important requisite later in life in using a barrier type of birth control, like a diaphragm or sponge. To minimize the potential of contracting toxic shock syndrome, I advise girls to use tampons only during the day, making sure to change them three to six times daily, depending on the volume of their menstrual flow, and to use sanitary pads at night. One final word on menstruation: Don't forget to demonstrate how to discard the product properly if you want to avoid costly plumbing bills or moments of unnecessary embarrassment.

Preparing daughters for this special event should be a joyful learning, laughing, giggling, and hugging experience. You might choose to make the occasion a true celebration. The event deserves to be heralded!

Recently a parent shared a wonderful occasion that had occurred in her life. Her daughter had gotten her first period. The mother had been preparing for the event for years. She was determined that it would be a celebration. And so it was! Her daughter was at school at the time. Since her daughter's breasts were budding and she was developing pubic hair, both mother and daughter knew that the big event would soon arrive. Her daughter kept a small box of sanitary napkins in her locker—just in case. Her daughter handled the event skillfully. She called home to tell Mom the good news. Mom was waiting at school at 2 P.M. dismissal with hugs and kisses and a gold friendship ring welcoming her daughter into the fold of womanhood. Her daughter intends to give the ring to *her* daughter someday; this rite of passage will become a family tradition.

Today, the rise in the number of single parents has resulted in parents of the opposite sex frequently being asked to assist their child with important facts about body changes. If you are speaking to your child of the opposite sex, or even of the same sex, consider the following true story.

I'll always remember the day when I, a preteen, was at the beach with a group of boys and girls. One of the boys commented that the chocolate ice cream I had been eating had dripped on my yellow bathing suit in a most inappropriate place. Everyone looked at my crotch and laughed. I ran to the ocean to wash away the brown stain, only to find that it reappeared again, but that this time it looked red—like blood. I clearly remember panicking, thinking that I was hurt and bleeding from this weird place in my body. A more experienced friend took me aside and sensitively explained what had happened. I wrapped a towel around my waist and went to my friend's home for menstrual first-aid. Later, when relating this most embarrassing moment to my mother, she was surprised that I had been so mystified. After all, she had given me a book to read about menstruation. She had felt sure that I knew everything there was to know. I never remember reading the book, but I do remember that it was left on my night table some months prior to the event. I may have glanced at it, but it looked too technical. When my mother asked if I had any questions about the information, I said "No"; therefore, she felt that I had understood it all.

My mother was on the right track in attempting to prepare me for the upcoming event. But a book alone, without the guidance and dialogue of a wiser, older person, is of little value. Parents often tell me that they have educated their children about sexuality. However, their child may confide that her parents have never talked to her about sex. Either the parent gave the child educational literature and the child claimed (as I had when questioned) that she understood it all, or the parent glossed over the subject in an awkward, haphazard way. Teen/parent sexuality studies bear out the fact that *both parents and children wish they could have dialogue with one another about sex.* Significantly, parents often believe that they have had such discussions, while less than one-third of the teens remember this happening. Subjects such as menstruation, first ejaculation, and nocturnal orgasms are rarely discussed. If they are, it is usually *after* the event has occurred. One day too late is nearly as remiss as not at all.

While I urge you to speak to your daughter about menstruation before the event occurs (when her breasts begin to develop), I also must share with you the consequences of giving *too much* information too soon. As our daughter approached puberty, I put my sex-educator skills into action. I explained the function of the reproductive organs, using diagrams and a pelvic model. But every time I tried to explain the biological details, Debbie became fidgety and uninterested. "Tell me about when you got your period" was really all she wanted to know.

Even though I couldn't seem to spark enthusiasm about the menstrual cycle, I continued to broach the subject with a positive attitude. I assured Debbie that we would celebrate the event when it occurred.

Months later, I received a call in my office. Debbie spoke in muffled tones. Her hand was cupping the telephone so no one in the school hallway would hear. "I got it!" she said. I was distracted and could hardly hear what she was saying. "What?" I responded. "I got it," she said again. Now she was impatient and shouted into the phone. "You know, *It.* I got *It!*" I couldn't help but laugh as the tears welled in my eyes. My baby had gotten her first period. "I'm so happy for you!" I exclaimed. "Do you have the sanitary napkins I gave you to keep in your locker?" "No," she said, "my friends used them a long time ago." "OK, go to the school nurse; she'll help you." "Don't worry, Mom, it won't be a problem," Debbie replied. "I'm not at the beach in a yellow bathing suit. I'll just stuff my pants with tissues. I'll be OK till I get home. The real reason that I am calling," she continued, "is about that celebration that you talked about. Will we have it tonight? Will we have a cake? Will everyone buy me a present?"

Here I was, the sex educator who had told her daughter everything she needed to know. But what had she remembered? Not the joyful journey of the ovum, but the possibility of a great celebration! Our daughter, now 21, recently told me that it was my personal account that really had prepared her for the Big Day.

For the single father raising his daughter without the aid of a mother, I recommend that you explain to a significant woman friend in your life that you need a first-person account of a menarche experience so that you can prepare your daughter with facts and feelings. Women are usually delighted to share this first experience and will give you insights about the sensitive side of becoming a woman. You could use my story, but it's always better when the child can relate the account to a woman she knows. Your next step is to create a Golden Opportunity, perhaps akin to the one here.

✳ ✳ ✳ You and your daughter are leafing through a magazine, and you come across an advertisement for sanitary products. Or, you pick up your daughter's teen magazine and call her attention to an ad. Or, you are watching TV and one of those ethereal commercial messages that euphemistically refer to the menses as "those delicate days" flashes across the screen. Or, you are shopping in the supermarket and you comment on the array and display of sanitary products. You say (if you're in the supermarket), "Remind me to tell you in the car an interesting (or funny) story that Jane Smith (Aunt Sue) told me about the first time she got her period." If you

> are at home, comment on the advertisement and then nonchalantly relate Jane's story as you would any story about a natural everyday experience.

You can show your daughter that, since speaking to Jane Smith you have bought some sanitary pads just to have them in the house when the occasion arises. Remind your daughter that you used to be a Boy Scout and you know the virtues of being prepared. Open the box and ask your daughter to help you figure out from the instructions how the products work. Keep the patter light and lively. After all, if Jane Smith (Aunt Sue) has told you about her first experience, it must not be such a secret subject. And if she has given you permission to share her story with your daughter, certainly there should be no embarrassment. After all, you are only talking about women doing what comes naturally.

I must share one final anecdote related to me by Roger, a delightful 63-year-old grandfather. He and his 12-year-old granddaughter Melissa went on a camping trip. They were just getting ready to throw their freshly caught fish on the fire when Roger's granddaughter discovered she was bleeding from her vagina. Melissa revealed the event by saying in a coquettish fashion, "I don't know how to tell you this, Popi, but I just got my first period." Roger told me: "We both looked at each other and laughed. I felt so damn strange. First of all, Melissa and I do so many things together that I don't often think of her as a girl. Second, I never thought to prepare myself for such an event to occur at a remote campsite! I told Melissa that I might be able to teach her a lot about fishing and camping, but that when it comes to women's stuff, I felt like a fool. I told her that I had been so dumb about girls as a kid that I had actually thought that when a girl didn't wear lipstick to school, it meant that she had her period.

"I also revealed a secret I had never told to anyone before. When I was growing up, I asked my mom what was in the little packages she used to throw away in the bathroom wastebasket. She told me it was a 'gift from God.' I couldn't understand why Mom would discard a gift from God, so one day I took one of these packages into my room to explore the contents of this so-called gift.

I nearly fainted when the unwrapped gift revealed a blood-stained gauze pad. It must be a blood-offering, I thought, like you read about in the Bible. It took me months to find the courage to get the inside story from my mother."

Melissa and Roger did a lot of laughing and serious talking that night. Melissa reassured her grandfather that she knew the basics about menstruation from school and her friends. Roger and Melissa fashioned sanitary pads from cotton batting and large gauze squares in the first-aid kit. Melissa and her grandfather had never felt closer as they imagined what Indian women and backwoods women had used as sanitary devices.

Roger revealed nearly forgotten memories of his adolescence that were triggered by this special event. They sat around the fire talking about kissing, dating, petting, and drive-in movies. "I even told her some locker room secrets, like how guys feel about their penises and 'circle jerks' (when guys sit in a circle and masturbate). Then I mentioned the sure-fire lines that boys have been using for years to seduce girls into having sex." Roger was misty-eyed as he ended our conversation, stating, "That was one very special camping trip!"

RITES OF PASSAGE: BOYS WILL BE MEN

While a girl's ascent to womanhood is dramatic, a boy's claim to manhood is less well defined. Some believe that it occurs at the time of a ceremonial bath, religious confirmation, the first orgasmic experience, or the first episode of sexual intercourse. In some cultures, the ritual of entering manhood is enacted through the surgical removal of the thin, loose skin (foreskin) that covers the head of the penis. In some cultures, this circumcision is performed when a boy reaches adolescence. For the Moslems, it occurs before puberty; for the Jews, it must be performed on the eighth day of life. More than one million babies in the United States are circumcised every year at their parents' request, for religious, ritual, or hygienic reasons.

IT'S WHAT'S UP FRONT THAT COUNTS: CIRCUMCISION

In all their married years, Sally and Craig had had no religious conflicts—until their son Daniel was born. Sally's Jewish faith insists that her son be circumcised in order to fulfill Abraham's covenant with God, as set forth in the book of Genesis. As a physician, Craig thought that the ritual was psychologically and medically traumatic for an infant. He believed that Daniel could easily learn to clean the secretions that accumulate under the foreskin (smegma) and therefore eliminate the chance of infection. Craig also concurred with modern thought that there is no real evidence that a circumcised penis is a deterrent to penile cancer or to the development of female cervical cancer.

Craig produced research for Sally to study that disputed her time-honored belief that circumcised men have greater penile sensitivity and greater ejaculatory control. In fact, the findings showed that there were no benefits to circumcision other than fulfilling an act of faith. For three days after Daniel's birth, Sally and Craig's joy was marred by their unrelenting commitment to opposing views. "He won't look like you" and "He'll look different from other boys," Sally argued. "Women don't like to make love to a man with an uncircumcised penis." Craig countered, "There are millions of uncircumcised men who have no trouble finding women."

Finally, the great debate was called to a halt. It appeared that proponents of each school of thought had equally convincing arguments to substantiate their point of view. For each study affirming increased body pride and sexual satisfaction, there was another study disclaiming the findings. The same held true for the medical implications—except for a recent study from the Center for Disease Control in Atlanta, Georgia, proposing that a circumcised penis is less apt to harbor bacteria and viruses, under the foreskin, especially the virus of AIDS. While Sally was not eager to subject her baby to a surgical procedure, she was also influenced by the possibility of further traumatizing her child if there was a need or a desire for a circumcision later. Above all, her religion dictated that she answer to a higher authority. On day eight, Daniel received his rite of passage.

Is circumcision necessary? Several schools of thought hotly debate the issue. One school believes that the body is a perfect package. As we continue to learn more about the body, these proponents say, we will find that the foreskin has a distinct and beneficial purpose. The other school of thought is that the foreskin serves no purpose other than as a source of infection. In light of the variety of lovemaking styles, why maintain a flap of skin that may harbor sexually transmitted disease? Another school of thought believes that the nerve endings found in the foreskin heighten a man's sexual excitement. They argue that the circumcised penis is less sensitive because the exposed head or glans is toughened by its proximity to clothing. That argument is countered with the notion that if the penis is less sensitive, a man will therefore develop better ejaculatory control.

Before Sally made her final decision in favor of circumcision, she consulted with friends. Their responses were equally divided. One mother stated that she found it time-consuming to clean her son, especially after he had a bowel movement. Another mother stated that she thought the act was barbaric and she couldn't bear the thought of it. An older male friend said that as a child he had been bothered with infections because his foreskin was so tight (phimosis) that he had had difficulty pulling it back for cleaning. He was circumcised when he was nine years old and had had nightmares for a while about his penis being cut off. Another circumcised male friend said he was surprised the first time his stepbrother revealed his uncircumcised penis but that aside from teasing each other about whose looked better, there really was no difference.

Sally confessed that she had mixed feelings about discussing her infant son's potential for sexual fulfillment. She wanted Daniel to feel proud of his penis, and she surprised herself in particularly being concerned (and later relieved) to learn that the removal of the foreskin would not diminish Daniel's ability to pleasure himself. Yet, she was embarrassed to admit that a major consideration in favor of a circumcision was that Daniel's desirability as an adult partner engaging in oral sex might be increased. "It's one thing to talk about being sexually liberated, but it is a very different matter to envision your baby as a sexually active adult," she said. Another lesson Sally learned was that such thinking in relation to an infant daughter seemed even more defiling. Some place deep in her heart she could reconcile Daniel's sexuality, but the only thought that came to mind in relation to a girl was "not with my daughter, you don't!" The circumcision issue was a rude awakening to the fact that a child's sexual health is central to his or her total happiness.

BODY TALK:
A BOY AND HIS ANATOMY

Judith is a 41-year-old pregnant single woman who selected a male partner to act as a sperm donor. She desperately wanted to have a child, but refused to marry in a rush just to fulfill her desire. Now five months pregnant, she has discovered by amniocentesis that she will deliver a healthy baby boy. She had secretly yearned for a girl, thinking it would be easier as a single woman to raise a daughter. Now she is emotionally preparing herself to address some of the anticipated sexual concerns that may arise, such as nudity and role identification.

Judy has come to me, as she put it, "to learn about the nuts and bolts of male sexuality." I explain that males and females both share, to a different degree, the same hormones, estrogen, progesterone, and testosterone, but that it is the male hormone testosterone, secreted from the testes, that regulates pubic hair growth, shoulder and chest development, voice change, and growth of the testes and penis. The testes, or testicles, are to testosterone, sperm development, and nocturnal emission what the ovaries are to estrogen, progesterone, ovum development, and menstruation. We discuss how the adrenal, pituitary, parathyroid, pineal, and thymus glands and a portion of the pancreas interplay in sexual development.

Nature, in its infinite wisdom, designed our bodies to best accommodate its needs. The sperm, which are extremely sensitive to heat, will survive only in temperatures lower than the 98.6° temperature of the body. Therefore, the scrotum, which contains the testicles that store the sperm, are exposed to the cooler temperature outside the body. (See diagram of male anatomy in the Appendix.) In contrast, the ova (eggs), which require the warmth of the body temperature, are stored within the ovaries inside the woman's abdominal cavity. Sperm are so sensitive that they may not reproduce if they are exposed to the continuous heat of a hot tub. They may also be reduced by the heat generated by tight underwear.

At puberty, the penis takes on its role as a sexual organ to conduct the sperm from the testicles, through the sperm ducts (vas deferens), and out the urethra. Along the way, other fluids are picked up from the seminal vesicles, prostate gland, and cowpers gland, all of which create the sticky white discharge known as semen, or ejaculate, or "cum." In order for the ejaculate to be expelled out of the body, the penis becomes engorged with blood, to assist the muscles in expelling the fluid through the enlarged penis. The ejaculation of this fluid out of the body can occur as a result of a "wet dream," masturbation, or sexual intercourse.

As Judy began to feel more comfortable with "boy talk," I explained that for the first two years of life, there are more similarities than differences between girls and boys. During those first two years, Judy can dramatically influence her son's sexuality by conveying her values and attitudes about sexuality. I asked Judy to write a letter to her forthcoming son conveying Judy's best intentions for raising a sexually healthy child. The next week Judy completed her assignment.

A MOTHER'S LETTER OF LOVE

✳ ✳ ✳*Dear Son:* I am very new at this mothering business, but I am determined to do it to the best of my capabilities. I know that I am on the right road to assist you in developing into a sexually healthy adult.

I have decided that I will shower with you and dress and undress in your presence until such a time that I feel uncomfortable, probably by the time that you are five years old. During these early years, I will explain the differences between our anatomy, using drawings and photographs to help in the discussions. I will also keep a keen eye out for Golden Opportunities, which are becoming more obvious to me as I look to nature and everyday occurrences.

To help you establish a healthy male identity, I am collecting promises from some of the men in my life. Uncle Mark promises to teach you how to swim, and Cousin Neal will take you to his photography studio. When it comes to thorny issues such as masturbation and wet dreams, I will clearly state my feelings, just as I would if I were raising a daughter. I approve of pleasuring yourself in a private setting. I will tell you that most of my male friends have had wet dreams and that my friends have told me that the release of semen, which some people call "cum" or "ejaculation," just happens involuntarily, like a sneeze or cough.

I will tell you that many of my friends have said that sometimes they have sexual dreams about people they know, but that's OK and normal. Dreams are only thoughts; they do not harm anybody. I will tell you that dreams are often about people you know only because your mind is familiar with those faces and that you need never act upon these dreams when you are awake. I will prepare you for your first wet dream before puberty, probably when you're seven or eight. I will herald its arrival as your initiation into manhood; similar to my first period. I'll assure you that the sheets can be washed easily and that it will not become a problem for anyone, most importantly not for you.

I am counting the days until I can hold you in my arms. I can hardly wait to share with you my knowledge and love!

Judy recognized that she may not have all the answers, but she is not concerned. She has identified friends, family, a trusted physician and sexuality counselor whom she may consult. Her support system for raising a sexually healthy child is firmly in place.

WET DREAMS: A STICKY SUBJECT

In my sexuality seminars, many men recall that there was no help from home to allay the confusion they felt as their pubescent body displayed its sexual changes. They felt the need to communicate that confusion at ages 11, 12, and 13. Sadly, for many, that need has continued into manhood.

Frequently I ask men these questions:

- Do you remember your first wet dream?
- Did you conceal the sticky sheets?
- Did you tell Mom that the dog "wet on the bed" or that you had spilled a glass of milk on the sheet?
- Were you frightened or delighted?

How reassuring it would have been for men to have been told that the nocturnal release of semen was a totally involuntary phenomenon. The fantasies associated with wet dreams may portray forbidden behavior, but many men don't understand that this is normal. Fantasies are rarely acted out during waking hours. In fact, fantasies are encouraged by health educators; fantasies are an alternative to intercourse as a form of safe sex.

Some men who choose to masturbate to release semen may never have a wet dream. In the beginning, the ejaculate may not yet contain sperm cells, so the fluid released is primarily from the prostate gland. The sperm, some 200 to 600 million per ejaculate, make up a small proportion of the total volume of semen. No matter how many times you ejaculate, you never can use up all of your sperm. The amount and consistency of ejaculate varies for each person and may be different for the same man from time to time. Sometimes it is thick and sticky, at other times it is thin and watery. The amount of seminal fluid in an ejaculation is approximately one and one-third teaspoon. Generations of boys would have been relieved to learn that, although an erection may be called a "boner," the penis is spongy and there is no bone within that will break. The size of the penis is not related to a man's body build or his ability to satisfy a sexual partner. (The average length of an adult's penis is between three and four inches when flaccid, increasing to five or seven inches when erect.) Think of the boys (and girls, too) who would have breathed easier knowing that they would not be sore or develop "blue balls" if they did not ejaculate every time their penis got hard. Wouldn't they rather have known that orgasm and ejaculation are two different things, and one does not have to follow the other in order for the individual to be normal and healthy? After all, before puberty, a boy could have hundreds of orgasms without ejaculating. A grown man may also have nonejaculatory orgasms even though he is producing sperm and will continue to produce sperm until the day he dies. Some men experience a series of orgasms without ejaculating and then ejaculate at the final orgasm.

In short, an orgasm is what a person *feels* and ejaculation is what a person *does*. A person can have one without the other. That's OK and natural. Both boys and girls are orgasmic, but girls do not ejaculate. The vagina becomes moist with small drops of liquid during sexual excitement. Girls, although less frequently, may also have orgasms in their sleep.

The first ejaculation (spermache) usually occurs between ages 11 to 16, after a boy's testicles and penis begin to increase in size and pubic hair appears at the base of the penis. This is the time for Dad, if he is available, to share a favorite boy-to-man experience. Unfortunately, in many homes there are no men to share this sexual history with their son. Divorce, as well as personal choice, has resulted in an increasing number of single parents.

I suggest that single mothers follow the advice that I have outlined for single fathers in the previous section on menstruation. Ask a close male friend or relative to relate his memories of his first wet dream. You might find that he is initially surprised by your request, but when you explain your need he'll probably be delighted to assist. Ideally, a parent educates herself in advance of a child's need, as Judy has done. Sexuality education is an ongoing process; it doesn't begin with the first nocturnal emission.

Felicia is the single parent of 11-year-old Geoffrey. She has never spoken to Geoffrey about sexual issues. She hopes he is learning everything he needs to know at school. In her quest to find male companionship for Geoffrey, Felicia enrolls him in Little

League. After the first day's practice, a Golden Opportunity presents itself. Geoffrey has been told that he needs a physical exam along with a list of required equipment, including an athletic supporter.

✳ ✳ ✳ "I see you need an athletic supporter," Felicia comments. "Yes," Geoffrey proudly responds. "What is an athletic supporter?" Felicia queries. "I don't know," Geoffrey shrugs. "All I know is that it's supposed to protect your jewels." "What jewels?" Felicia naïvely counters. "My jewels! You know, my nuts!" Felicia tells Geoffrey that she's been meaning to talk to him about the way his body is changing, but she is not sure about the way a boy's body works. Felicia asks Geoffrey for assistance. Geoffrey, feeling very important that he knows more about sex than Mom, agrees to help her learn. On the way home they stop at the library and borrow some books on adolescent sexuality. Geoffrey, who is a fair to poor student, can hardly wait to get home and read! Felicia and Geoffrey leaf through one book containing many pictures, nonchalantly glancing at a picture of a penis, a vulva, and breasts. Their initial impulse to laugh is quelled as Geoffrey and Mom begin to examine this important information. "Look," Geoffrey exclaims, "there's a picture of an athletic supporter. I told you it was supposed to protect your jewels. It says 'the scrotum has been referred to as "the jewels" because it's considered such an important part of a man's body.' And look what else it says about the testicles that are stored inside the scrotum: 'In ancient Rome men would cross their hands over their testicles when they made a promise, meaning that a man's word is as good as his testes.' Oh my gosh, that's where the word *testify* comes from!

"Wow," exlaims Geoffrey, pointing out another paragraph. "This explains why I can't find my balls— 'scuse me, Mom—my scrotum after I go swimming. They move inside your body when they get too cold and come down when the temperature is right. Every time I go swimming I get scared that my balls— 'scuse me, Mom—my scrotum, will disappear. You know what, Mom," Geoffrey suddenly confides, "the other night I thought I lost my scrotum when my penis got real hard and some white stuff came out of it. I thought the white stuff meant that I had touched something the wrong way and hurt something inside."

The time was right for Felicia to fill in all the gaps. Geoffrey desperately needed this information! If Felicia had simply bought the athletic strap without pursuing the questions, she would have remained unaskable, and Geoffrey would still be groping for answers. The lesson is:

- It's never too late to begin your child's sexuality education.
- Any parent can do a fine job if he or she is available, or "askable," in a loving and understanding manner.
- Keep your eyes open for Golden Opportunities. Sometimes they are in clear sight and you can't—or won't—see the signal.

Even in a two-parent household, a child may be hungering for information, yet his or her obvious behavior doesn't awaken the assistance of his parents.

Florence was accustomed to making her son Jason's bed every morning, even though she insisted that he should assume this responsibility and promised each day that this would be the last time she would be his housekeeper. You can imagine her surprise when Jason announced one day that he had made his bed and would continue to do so from then on! It was at this time that Jason also began to close his bedroom door at night and ask that nobody enter without knocking.

Florence and her husband David smiled knowingly. Jason, at 13, was discovering his manhood. But, they wondered, what actually went on behind the closed door? Although they were curious, neither parent felt ready or able to talk with Jason. One morning Florence met Jason in the laundry room with his bed linen. He was trying to figure out how to use the washing machine. Florence said that she would do the laundry and reached for the linen. Jason grabbed his linen possessively and in a shrill voice insisted upon doing his own laundry. An onlooker might have found the tug-of-war over the linen amusing if it hadn't been for the tears running down Jason's cheeks. Seeing them, Florence saw her Golden Opportunity.

✳ ✳ ✳Florence stopped tugging and began hugging Jason. "It's OK," she said. "I know all about it. It happens to all men and boys. Please don't be embarrassed. It's I who should be ashamed for not having the courage to talk with you sooner." She continued to hug Jason as she spoke. "Jason, nobody ever talked to Dad and me about sex when we were growing up, and most of what we learned from friends was wrong. Jason, you deserve better. We'll get some books from the library to look at together.

"I want you to know that whatever you are experiencing and feeling is *normal*. Everyone passes through a state in life when hormones come alive. It takes time to get used to the changes that your body is feeling. If you are waking with an erection, it's normal. If you have a dream at night and your penis gets hard and ejaculates white creamy fluid, it's normal. If you are concerned about the size of your penis as you compare it to others', it's normal. It's all normal! Your dad had the same concerns when he was a teenager and he has survived. Every man has felt as you feel now—your teacher, your uncles, the gardener, the postman, even our pastor."

Florence's hug loosened and Jason's tears evaporated. The chance meeting in the laundry room was an experience that never could have been planned. It was a Golden Opportunity just waiting to be discovered. Doesn't your son deserve better than you got? Of course he does. That's why you are reading this book. Sensitivity, honest disclosure, kindness, and good humor set the stage for boy-to-parent talks.

IS BIGGER BETTER?
A BOY AND HIS PENIS

Recently, two teenage boys entered my office with a camera and a notepad. Their school newspaper had assigned them to interview me about the current trends of teenage sexuality. In a businesslike manner, the interviewer queried me: "Why is the birth control pill the most popular form of contraception for teenage girls? What do you think of the contraceptive sponge, which can be bought over the counter without a doctor's prescription? If condoms are such reliable safeguards against sexually transmitted diseases and unplanned pregnancies, why is there such a controversy about advertising them through the media?"

The questions were good. As both boys prepared to leave, I sensed that one boy had some personal concerns. Sure enough, within five minutes he had returned, alone.

"Quick," he stated, "I need to ask you a few questions but I don't want my friend to know." He stammered and blushed and finally asked, "Is it true that bigger is better? How big is big enough?" He went on to say that he believed that his penis was undersized, judging from comparisons he had made with the boys in the locker room.

I explained that it is a myth that bigger is better. Couples, regardless of the size of the penis or length and width of the vagina, adjust their lovemaking style to accommodate each other's unique packaging. I then pulled out a pelvic model and assured him that women also come in different vaginal lengths and widths, and that the elasticity of the vaginal wall enables it to adjust to almost any size penis. I explained that while men derive their greatest sexual excitement through the penis, women most enjoy clitoral pleasure and desire heightened sexual excitement within the first third of the vaginal canal. I reassured him that a flaccid penis is not an indicator of its size when it becomes erect. In fact, smaller-size penises become even larger when erect than larger-size ones. The average size penis is about six inches long when erect, but it's quite normal to be shorter, longer, thicker, or thinner than others and may even curve when erect.

"Wow, what a relief! Can I call you if I need help again? You see," he continued, "I'm still a virgin, and from the way my friends talk I guess I'm the last one around. I've been afraid that I wasn't big enough to please a woman. Besides, almost every girl has had sex, and I'm afraid they will know more about it than I do."

"On the contrary," I countered, "I meet many virgins every day. It is not going out of style. All boys tend to brag. I'd be willing to bet that many of your friends are in the same place as you are. As for having sex with a so-called "experienced woman," I wouldn't think that being a virgin on such an occasion would be a source of embarrassment. In fact, it is a wonderful compliment to a future partner that you have decided to wait for just the right person with whom to share this special encounter. I believe a woman would feel flattered. I also suggest that you choose wisely, because you are a very special young man."

LOCKER ROOM AND BATHROOM POLITICS

Many boys I counsel say that they've learned almost everything they need to know about sex from the boys' locker room. Open shower stalls and urinals give them an opportunity to view each other from head to toe.

This viewing becomes the measure by which a boy compares his height, weight, muscle strength, and the size and shape of his genitals. It may be a cause for panic if a child's body clock dictates a slow growth rate while a locker partner boasts large muscles and a well-developed penis. Clearly, if bigger is better, vast numbers of boys begin to devalue their maleness at an early age.

For girls who suffer through communal showers feeling under-developed or overly endowed or ashamed if one breast is larger than the other (which is normal, but few girls know this), the emotional pain may be equally devastating.

While there appears to be an insensitive attitude about nudity in the boys' locker room, we might assume that the privacy doctrine used for girls' bathrooms would eliminate self-doubt. Yet this is not the case.

Early in life, females are taught bathroom etiquette: Never use a dirty facility, always "paper the seat," so your skin doesn't touch where another's skin has been. Lock the door securely. Wads of paper must be used to protect hands from accidentally touching genitals. Always wash hands thoroughly before leaving the bathroom.

Girls get the message that everything from the waist down is dirty, untouchable, and not to be viewed by others, except perhaps by a doctor or husband. Certainly this area is not to be examined by its owner.

In contrast, boys are programmed to shower freely and to touch and expose their bodies, like it or not. After all, "it's only normal."

Normal? Not for most of the men whom I have met in counseling. They have confided that they never felt comfortable about their body shape and their penis size. They wished someone had explained in their youth that each person is packaged distinctly and that size does not reflect one's ability to be "all male." These men remember cowering in a corner of the locker room, embarrassed to expose themselves to peers. Some remember pretending to have a chill so that they would not have to expose their chests at the beach.

These men had no loving teachers to assure them that their adolescent breast development was normal and that exercise and maturity would transform this fatty tissue into toned muscle. No one ever told them that the body is not a symmetrical form and that if a chalk line were drawn from the head to the toes, one easily would see that one eye is larger than the other and that the same holds true for one nostril, one breast, one teste (usually the left), and even one foot. A shoe size is a good analogy that everyone can relate to without embarrassment. Girls benefit from this explanation as well and often breathe a sigh of relief in knowing that nobody's body is a symmetrical creation. In fact, the body is as customized as a person's thumbprint.

Daughters must be reassured that they may touch their bodies without a sense of shame and disgust. If for no other reason, they must learn this to perform breast self-exam, to insert vaginal hygiene products, and, of course, to use contraceptive controls such as the diaphragm.

Sons need to learn by example that men can talk to one another, not as competitors, but as friends who have fears and doubts about their bodies and their budding sexuality. True friends need not brag; true lovers need not fake it. True men need not maintain a macho facade.

I have counseled men who were so stigmatized by the locker room politics as children that today they have developed what is known as a "bashful kidney." It is a condition where they strategize their entire day's schedule to avoid the necessity of having to urinate in the open stall of a public restroom. In fact, they *cannot* urinate in such a setting.

We are unable to change bathroom and locker room etiquette outside the home, but perhaps inside the home we can initiate change by affirming the beauty of being similar to, but not exactly like, another. Respecting one's sense of modesty and privacy as well as respecting one another's differences is what we hope to achieve.

But how do you begin to initiate change at home if you still grapple with unhappy locker room memories? Perhaps you are a woman who cowers in the corner of a department store dressing room or a man who refuses to join the gym because of the communal showers. You may doubt your ability to convey healthy messages to your children when you have not resolved your own inhibitions.

GOLDEN OPPORTUNITIES FOR THE SEDATE TO THE ADVENTUROUS

Perhaps you can begin to erase your own doubts and uncertainties by participating in the Golden Opportunities described here. Some of the suggestions may sound intimidating at first. Always proceed at your own speed, using your sense of comfort as a measure of when to take the next step.

1. A mirror will bring you face to face with your best friend—yourself. Make it a point to look at yourself whenever the opportunity arises. In the privacy of your home, slowly examine your facial features as you smile, frown, and laugh. Watch how you look as you speak. Gradually focus on other parts of your body until you feel at ease viewing all of you in a dressed and undressed state. Decide which parts of your body you find most attractive and then decide how to become less critical of the areas you find least attractive. Exercise, diet, improved posture, cosmetics, flattering clothing, and even cosmetic surgery may revise your perception. Do keep in mind that few people look like media idols. *It is the uniqueness of each body that makes each of us recallable to others.*

2. Next time you shower or bathe, take the time to experience the feel of your body. Slowly soap your skin and allow yourself to absorb the sensuous pleasures derived from touch. An oil-scented bath, finished with a warm towel wrap, is a simple way to increase the appreciation of your custom-made body. You may discover a mole on your left leg. You may feel giggly as you wash between your toes or a warm glow when you wash under your arms. You may be surprised at the smoothness of your skin or may decide to remove a callus from the heel of your foot. There is a joy in claiming a sense of ownership of your body. The more

adventurous you become, the greater is the likelihood that you will begin to recognize the beauty of your body. It is also a safeguard in detecting any unusual lesions or irregular growths. If you feel stressed at the concept of self-examination, put this exercise aside. Do not feel pressured to do anything at any time that makes you feel uncomfortable. Maybe you'll choose to reconsider the prospect at a later time, maybe not. Either way, it's OK. The most important thing is to *be kind and patient with yourself, and this will emerge in how you deal with your children as well.*

3. If you feel adventurous, try this exercise: In the privacy of your home, use a mirror to examine your genitals. If you are female, you may now locate your vulva, with its labia, clitoris, urethra and the mouth of the vagina. You may wish to use the anatomical drawings in the Appendix to find each part. Braver women may progress to using a speculum to open the walls of the vagina, and a mirror and flashlight to look inside. Actually, this kind of close examination is not an unusual procedure. Advanced methods of natural family planning require that women check their vaginal secretions at each phase of the monthly cycle to know when the secretions will be most hostile or receptive to receiving sperm.

If you are male, use a flashlight and mirror to examine your scrotum and testes and locate your vas deferens, epididymis, and spermatic cord. There is a male anatomical drawing in the Appendix with definitions and locations. Such exams are highly recommended by theorists who believe that the better you know your body, the more apt you are to maintain its healthy status.

4. As you begin to better know yourself, look more carefully at others at the beach, gym, and neighborhood pool. Everywhere you go there are opportunities to people-watch. Notice the different sizes and shapes in which people come packaged. Notice how few people look like movie stars. Notice how many bodies are coupled with bodies that seem so ill matched. Notice that attraction is in the eye of the beholder and that each person obviously is attracted to another because of *a personal perception of beauty.*

5. As you begin to appreciate the wonders of you, treat yourself to a therapeutic body massage. Join a fitness club or treat yourself to a few days at a spa. Notice the array of body shapes in the exercise room and dressing room. Notice how nonchalant the people are in dressing and undressing. Notice someone who appears to be comfortable and try to emulate that person's actions.

I hope that these exercises will help you overcome unpleasant memories of the past. In becoming your own best friend, you show your children that the body is to be cared for and valued. You will probably discover that your sense of pride is contagious. It will be reflected in the heightened enjoyment and comfort you show in assisting your children to become sexually healthy adults.

$$*7*$$

Friends and Relationships

Chapter 6 opened with secrets disclosed by special friends at a slumber party. Friendships at all ages affirm our sense of worth and acceptance. Did you ever have a special best friend with whom you shared secrets about your parents, your body and the way it was changing, your first menstruation or wet dream, your first kiss, or your first sexual encounter?

FRIENDS AS MEASURES OF SEXUAL IDENTITY

As children grow, their need for friendship increases. This is a time for separating from parents, for spending the day at someone else's house, for watching how friends relate to their families. It means day care, schools, playgrounds, and sleep-over dates.

In these activities, children learn the benefits of giving and taking, of sharing and guarding possessions. These same elements will be called into play as their childhood friendships mature into adult intimacies. These separate the sensitive, considerate lover in later life from the aggressive, self-centered sexual partner.

Randy and Scott are playing baseball. Randy owns the bat and ball. Randy refuses to play by the rules, which makes Scott very angry. What are Scott's alternatives?

Here is a Golden Opportunity in the making. Healthy friendships, like healthy sexual relationships, require special skills. In this instance, Scott's mother suggests a technique for helping Scott hypothesize his alternatives. The process is similar to the "What if" games played in early childhood. Scott's mother asks Scott to think through what can happen if one decision is selected as opposed to what can happen if an alternative is chosen. At one end of the continuum is "the worst thing that can happen." At the other extreme is "the best thing that can happen." Somewhere in the middle lies the realistic alternative—usually a compromise between both extremes.

Scott decides to talk to Randy. After all, "what's the worst thing that could happen?" Randy could hit Scott over the head with his bat and go home. The best thing that could happen is that Randy will correct his ways and even thank Scott for bringing this deficit to his attention. What's likely to happen if Scott expresses his feelings with kindness? Randy may begin to play by the rules. If Scott remembers to compliment Randy each time he cooperates, perhaps Randy will remember that it feels nice to be nice.

This episode seems unrelated to love and sex. But think of what an important role it plays for adults who need to resolve conflict. Randy shows the same aggressive traits that many adults complain about in discussing their partner's excessive sexual demands. Many partners are unable to state the rules for intimacy clearly. One party feels abused and resents the other party, who cares only about having his or her needs met: "If you don't have sex with me, I'll take my bat and ball and go home." Sound familiar? It need not be, once you learn to communicate the rules for fair play.

For the first five or six years, children may play with peers of the opposite and same sex, but their greatest devotion is to their parents. As their bodies assume new shapes, and their feelings change, children look to one another as foils for an acceptable self-image (usually from ages 6 to 12). It's a normal time for healthy children to turn away from their parents.

They may even become critical and argumentative, believing that their parents do not display behavior that inspires peer recognition. Close friendships at this age are usually with friends of the same sex. Children often form clubs with secret rituals, oaths of loyalty, and unintelligible languages to preserve their privacy. Everyone has the need for privacy, and certainly this need should be respected. After all, have you told your parents *everything* that occurred in your life? This reality in no way diminishes the love you feel for your parents, any more than it will threaten your parent-child relationship.

Like adolescence, it's an age when a child plays sex games, masturbates, and has crushes on people, but at this time, it is directed to people of the same sex. Parents often become concerned that this behavior forecasts a lifelong behavior pattern when, in fact, it is a transitory stage that helps children rehearse for heterosexual relationships. "Am I normal?" is the underlying concern. Their need to be alike is intense, because to look different is to jeopardize their acceptability to their peers. "Different" may mean being too tall, too short, too smart, or too dumb. Thus they copy each other's dress, hairstyle, jargon, and behavior. The struggle for acceptance is particularly poignant for the slow or precocious maturer.

I can recall one devastating incident that is indelibly recorded in my memory. A parent brought Alex, their 13-year-old son, to counseling. Alex had refused to attend school for over a week. More than a week before, Alex had celebrated his thirteenth birthday. He and his family had made elaborate plans to give Alex a lavish party. The finest caterer was hired. There was a band, flowers, party favors, and even a bus to pick up and deliver Alex's friends to and from the gala event. Two weeks before the gala, however, someone at school decided that Alex was a "fag." Maybe it was his white socks or his mathematical expertise or his strike-out at the bat. One by one, his classmates secretly decided to not attend Alex's party. Anyone attending the party would risk the wrath of "the group" and would be blackballed.

Alex's big day arrived. There were 200 adults at his party, but the elaborately decorated dais for 30 children was empty. The bus arrived, but there was no one on board. There was no happiness in Alex's heart despite the loving family, the music, and the gifts. He spent the next week locked in his room refusing to eat and begging to be left alone.

How can one measure the insult to Alex's identity? Such a cruel, premeditated act of rejection can leave scars that probably will never heal completely. I often tell this true story when I teach sexuality to early adolescents. I dramatize every aspect of the incident and then ask for a volunteer from the class to play the part of

Alex. You can feel the tension as each child rejects the request. "How would you feel if you were Alex?" I ask. "Who is to blame for this rejection?" The children vow that they will never perpetuate such an unkindness. "After all, I would never want anyone to do it to me," a child confirms. As to who is at fault, the children usually lay blame on Alex's so-called friends. I tend to hold the parents responsible for this hardship. Certainly, one parent should have had the kindness to insist that his or her child honor the promise to attend. Couldn't a parent have intervened by calling and informing the other parents of their children's secret plan?

Self-esteem is a fragile, precious quality that must be respected and preserved. The following is an easily adaptable Golden Opportunity to address the ridicule and meanness that is so prevalent during preadolescence.

✳ ✳ ✳ The principal of a local private school asked if I could offer a class that would address the unmerciful teasing that was taking place among the sixth-graders. The principal assumed it was related to the children's blossoming sexuality. She was right. The following week I brought to class a large bag of oak leaves. I asked each student to pick a leaf from the bag. "Now," I advised, "examine the leaf as you would a most precious possession. Touch it. Smell it. Observe every vein, every gradation of color." Some minutes later I collected the leaves (a few children protested, not wanting to relinquish this prized possession). I then dropped the leaves in a heap on the floor. (There were some complaints and consternation that I was abusing their possession.) Then I asked four children at a time to retrieve their leaves from the pile. In less than five minutes, 25 students had made a positive identification of their leaf. "How did you separate your leaf from all the others?" I asked. "Mine is yellow-green on its right side." "Mine is broad near the base." "Mine has three veins overlapping one another." "So," I said, *it's the differences that make your leaf special.* It's not the sameness. Your leaf would be boring if it had no distinguishing characteristics. These leaves are just like you and me. What makes each of us special is our uniqueness—being small or tall or round-faced or freckle-faced. To have long hair, wiry hair, long legs, or big feet is to have an identity of your own. It's the differences that make you rememberable. *It's the differences that make you lovable.* You could distinguish your leaf in a flash from its natural beauty or differences (or some may say imperfections). You knew that this was the first, the last, the one and only leaf of its kind.

"What does that tell you about people?" I asked. "What makes you different and therefore special and distinct? How can you preserve your identity? Who has the right to abuse your specialness? How can we avoid diminishing one another's unique qualities?"

Each student insisted on taking his or her leaf home. I have since met children and parents who have told me that the leaf is preserved in wax paper, framed, and affixed to the refrigerator. The principal was delighted in the improved camaraderie of the students. The everyday opportunity of observing a leaf-laden tree can provide a Golden Opportunity for sexuality education.

PEER PRESSURES: PUSH-PULL FROM PARENTS AND FRIENDS

Do you remember your first special friend of the opposite sex? Perhaps you gradually were separated from one another by social activities that segregated girls from the boys, such as sports and clubs. Frequently children innocently seek the companionship of the opposite sex. Adults too often disallow the friendship because of their unfounded fears of sexual play, when actually these relationships are the natural efforts of children to rehearse their roles as sensitive adults.

Special friendships are an important part of growing up in which children find acceptance from the opposite sex while measuring the relationship against their own belief system. Yet friendship is not a substitute for parents' love or knowledge. And while children may commiserate over their parents' misjudgments, they still require, at this age, the security of knowing that they need to abide by carefully assigned parental guidelines. Even protesting children yearn for parents' caring guidance. Many times, the louder the child protests, the more urgent the need for assistance.

Sixteen-year-old Peter protests that he's the only kid who can't go to the party on Wednesday night. Can he help it that the party falls on the Wednesday before final exams? What's he going to tell the girl who asked him to go? What's he going to tell his friends? He slams doors and pouts, but his parents do not relent. Secretly, Peter is relieved. His parents are right that he'd rather score high on the test than score with his friends on this occasion. Peter does not lose face with his peers when he confides that *he* wants to go to the party, but that his parents are too strict to let him. The truth is that Peter didn't want to spend an evening with the girl who extended the invitation, but he didn't know how to say "No" without hurting her feelings.

It is when a parent is unapproachable as a confidant that a child may succumb to peer pressure. If Peter's parents hadn't intervened, Peter would have been swept away by the persuasion of his peers. He may have failed the exam and probably would have discovered that spending the evening with a girl he dislikes was not worth the sacrifice. Without parental support, children must learn by trial and error.

Learning by experience is powerful *only* if the child doesn't interpret a parent's relaxed attitude as a sign of no interest. Children look to their parents for guidance and support. The process starts in childhood when choosing between two flavors of ice cream or deciding whether or not to wear a raincoat. *Helping your children at an early age to choose wisely allows them to make wise decisions in your absence.*

Suppose, for example, that Peter's parents were out of town. Here is how Peter arrives at a decision: "The worst thing that could happen is that I will miss a great party and my friends may think I'm queer. But I know that there will be more great parties, and I also know that I am not queer. The best thing that can happen is that the party is postponed until Saturday and that Wendy, whom I secretly love, will ask me to be her date *and* I will get an A + on my exam! What probably will happen is that if I study I will improve my grade. I'll miss the party, but I won't have to spend the evening with Sue, who is conceited. And, afterward, I won't stay awake all night cramming for the exam." Peter declines the invitation assertively, stating that the test is an unwelcome priority that nonetheless demands his attention. His friends try to dissuade him from this decision, but Peter stands firm. His friends secretly admire and respect him for having the courage of his own convictions.

LEVELS OF RELATIONSHIPS: STRANGERS, FRIENDS, LOVERS

I find that children, as well as adults, get tripped up in defining the significant people in their lives. The little child says, "I let the groceryman kiss me on the mouth because he said we are good friends." The preschooler is led away by a "nice" lady who says she has a kitten in her car. The preadolescent says, "Melody isn't my friend anymore; she won't keep a secret." The adolescent says, "I'm giving my house key to Vincent so he can sleep here when his folks lock him out." The young adult says, "I slept with him because I thought he loved me."

- To whom do you lend a key to your home, your car, your safe deposit box?
- Whom do you kiss on the mouth, in the mouth, on the cheek, not at all?
- With whom do you share your bicycle, your pencil, your new blue jacket?
- To whom do you tell a secret, the state of the weather, the directions to your home, your religious convictions?
- With whom do you masturbate, share caresses, have intercourse?

The answers to these questions help children delineate the privileges extended within specific relationships. The preschooler will understand that the groceryman is an *acquaintance.* We never kiss an acquaintance on the mouth. We say "Hi" to an acquaintance and share only a limited amount of information about ourselves. The preschooler will learn that the lady is a *stranger* and that you never go anywhere with or accept any gifts from a stranger. The preadolescent will appreciate that Melody is a *friend,* but that you share secrets only with family or with a trusted best friend. The adolescent will recognize that the key to your home is not to be given to a *special friend,* even though you share intimate secrets with one another. The key to the house is reserved for family and perhaps for a special friend of whom the whole family approves. (The fact that Vincent's parents lock him out of his own home makes one think that he may not be a person who is responsible enough to be afforded this privilege.) The young adult will acknowledge that while she reserved intercourse for her most *intimate relationship,* her partner defined intimacy by another standard. It takes time for an intimate relationship to progress from that of stranger to acquaintance to friend to very special friend. The time is required so that each person proves his or her commitment to the relationship through words and actions. A truly committed relationship usually begins with a common interest, from which spring qualities such as trust, sincerity, loyalty, humor, patience, and understanding.

All through life we struggle with relationships. Little children soon learn that a smiling face and a kind word does not always mean that an adult may be trusted. There are strangers who disguise themselves as friends, and there are intimate friends who may be more deceitful than strangers. The preadolescent who develops a genuine love relationship with a friend of the same sex soon learns that these special feelings are frowned upon by society.

The disappointment and confusion about relationships escalates for late-blooming adolescents who feel abandoned by their special best friends while the latter pursue a new allegiance with the opposite sex. Teens struggle with the yes/no messages from every element of society. Yes, be popular! No, don't encourage very special friendships for fear that they may lead to premature intimacy. What's even more confusing is that intimate relationships must now be laboratory tested for dreaded diseases before they are legitimately pursued. In addition, it is difficult to explain the boundaries of relationships to children when strangers often come to your rescue and intimate relations shun you because of their jealousy, anger, or greed. We can only hope that the example we set will become a model for our children to recognize qualities of kindness, sincerity, trust, and love in others.

We are not experts, but we each keep trying to find out truth. We do need to define some guidelines so that children understand that:

- A *stranger* is a person about whom we know nothing (the man walking down the street).
- An *acquaintance* is a person we know by name and about whom we have limited information (the school bus driver).
- A *friend* is a person whose first and last name we know, as well as special information about his or her likes, dislikes, interests, and needs. We usually know the address and telephone number of friends, too. (Jill is a friend.)
- A *very special friend* is a person about whom we know more than we do about a friend and with whom we share more personal thoughts and feelings. Special friends may share certain toys and belongings. Sometimes, if we want, we kiss or hug special friends. (Billy and Aunt Joyce and Mr. Levy are special friends.)
- *Intimate friends* are people who know the most about you. You can tell them anything and they will understand and love you. You can tell them a secret and they will not betray you or tell your secret to anyone else. Mommy and Daddy, Grandma, and Dr. Taylor are intimate friends. Intimate friends kiss and hug (although not always, because you may not want to kiss and hug Dr. Taylor). Intimate friends can touch you on a private part, with your permission, when you take a bath or if you are hurt and need first aid. You should always say, "Don't do that" if *anyone* does something that makes you feel uncomfortable or unhappy. You should also tell Mommy or Daddy about this, because we don't like it when anyone makes you feel sad or funny inside.

Golden Opportunities abound for defining relationships. You and your child can play the "relationship game." It's lots of fun. Before or after meeting someone, you simply declare the person's status—friend, acquaintance, special friend, intimate friend. If you are in an airport or a setting that attracts many people, you can guess the person's occupation and decide if you'd like to include the person in any of the relationship categories. This exercise provides additional opportunities to play "What if." "What if that man in the black coat were to ask you to assist him to the restroom?" "What if that sweet old lady were to offer you candy?" "What if that girl sat next to that boy in the airplane? What do you think they would talk about?"

As children are exposed to new relationships, the message must be repeated and reinforced, as you can see in the following Golden Opportunity.

✳ ✳ ✳ Twelve-year-old Allison grows tired of waiting for her mom to pick her up at her friend's house. "Where do you live?" asks the pizza delivery boy who is making a delivery to her friend's home. Allison tells him. The driver says that he's on his way to that part of town and invites her to join him. Allison accepts, only to be greeted by Mom as Allison is about to climb into the pizza van. Mom apologizes for being late and for tempting Allison to be unwise in her judgment. Mom asks Allison if she knows the pizza boy. Allison says "No." Mom asks if it was a wise decision to accept a ride from a stranger even in light of Allison's impatience. Allison agrees that it was foolish. "What other alternatives did you have?" Mom asks. Allison thinks for a while and decides that she could have:

- Asked her friend's mother for a lift
- Called Mom's office to see how late she would be
- Called Aunt Gale to pick her up
- Called the house to see if Dad had arrived home earlier than usual
- Asked to stay with her friend until Mom arrived
- Borrowed money to take a cab home

Mom had options, too. Mom could have:

- Reprimanded Allison: "You should know better!"
- Called Allison names like "stupid" and "untrustworthy"
- Lashed out at the delivery boy: "How dare you! I'm going to report you to your boss."
- Given Allison the silent treatment
- Threatened Allison with an unrealistic punishment:

"You'll never be allowed to come to this friend's home again."
- Made Dad the disciplinarian: "Wait until your father finds out; he'll hit the roof!"

Instead, Mom did not overreact. First, she apologized for the part she had played in creating the dilemma. Then she repeated the safety rules she and Allison have discussed many times before. Allison's mother knows that each new situation presents new challenges. Education about sexuality must be updated as the child matures.

You can help your children sort out the challenges of relationships by providing anecdotes for them to analyze. Children of all ages are responsive to "What if" puzzles. These provide the opportunity to rehearse real-life dilemmas. The following is a "what if" that calls for a variety of decision-making skills:

Thirteen-year-old Beth is feeling awkward at a house party that everyone else seems to be enjoying. As she walks to the bathroom for the eighth time, Sal, a boy whom she knows only casually, asks her to dance. She's so flattered and nervous that she barely notices that he's dancing much closer than he should. When the next dance begins, Sal is kissing Beth's neck and moving his hand toward the front of her sweater. Beth is frightened, but afraid to say "No" because she doesn't want to make a scene. Besides, she thinks everyone else in the darkened room must be doing the same thing.

You may present this scenario to your son or daughter during a quiet moment at home, or offer it for discussion during the family dinner. Brainteaser questions may range from "Do you think parents should be home when kids have a party?" to "What kind of a guy is Sal?" and "What should Beth say?" Answering them will strengthen your child's skill in decision-making, assertiveness, withstanding peer pressure, relationship-building, and observing social amenities. Again and again the skills that have been nurtured in childhood are tested and challenged with each new stage of sexual maturation.

BECOMING AN "ASKABLE" PARENT

When a parent is available, unhurried, patient, and sensitive, a child will not be fearful that his or her concerns will be met with ridicule, anger, or embarrassment. This parent is "askable." This parent will safeguard the child from misinformation. This parent will break the tradition of the vast majority of children learning everything they know about life, sex, and love from their friends.

How about making your child your friend by sharing your childhood memories? Break out the cookies and ice cream, kick off your shoes and take the phone off the hook. Take a deep breath and let the words flow. Maybe you have some old photo albums or scrapbooks. A fragile faded flower from your first prom, a movie stub from your first date, or a special letter from the first heartthrob you ever kissed, yearbooks that spark memories of your adolescent joys and pains, or even a tattered book of matches that lit up many parentally unsanctioned cigarettes. Children delight in hearing about their parents' youthful ups, downs, and transgressions.

Remember, you're your child's friend now and not the final authority. Encourage your child to explore all avenues of thought, weighing the risks and the benefits of each. Your child will begin to find a balance between aggressive and adaptive behavior that is most comfortable and produces the greatest amount of happiness. This is truly a gift that keeps on giving.

A DIFFERENT KIND OF FRIENDSHIP: HOMOSEXUALITY

But what of the child who silently agonizes over his or her sexual preference? Yearning for advice but fearful of ridicule and abandonment, the child secretly searches for an understanding of why she or he prefers friends of the same sex.

As I explained in the beginning of this chapter, children between the ages of 6 and 12 enter and usually pass through a stage of same-sex friendships as preparation for entering the next phase of development, which is dominated by an interest in the opposite sex. They often engage in trial-and-error activities in order to adapt to the changes in their appearance and emotions. In the respect that it is not harmful, their action is similar to the innocent exploration of the curious preschooler playing doctor.

Once in a while, children become stuck at this juncture. While their friends progress to heterosexual activities, they flounder in the mire of their own confusion: "What's wrong with me? Why don't I have the urge to be with a person of the opposite sex? I must not be normal."

These children are desperately in need of factual information! They don't know where to turn. Parents are desperately in need as well. *They* don't know where to turn. *They* often want to reach out to their anguished child, but they do not have the factual information that their child seeks. What frequently happens is that parents deny their intuition that their child is in a sexual identity crisis. "It's only a phase," they say. In the meantime, the child may avoid all social functions, abandon interest in school, or become totally absorbed in academic activities as a distraction for personal conflict.

What *are* the facts? And most important, what is your attitude about same-sex relationships? Even if you felt comfortable with information about homosexuality, would you be able to convey it to a child in a nonjudgmental manner?

In your lifetime, I'm sure that you have met homosexuals whom you may have admired and others whom you found repugnant. (Note that the same holds true of heterosexuals.) Those homosexuals whom you admired *in no way affected your sexual preference,* any more than homosexual schoolteachers can coerce a child to follow their personal life-style. (Most studies confirm that by the age of three, children are usually able to label themselves as boys or girls. By the age of five or six, it is believed that a child's sexual identity is locked in place.)

Research has disclosed that there is no one dynamic of family life that predisposes a child's heterosexual or homosexual orientation. There is no supporting evidence that parents are responsible for their children's homosexuality. In fact, neither parental nor social influences seem to have much effect on sexual preference.

Some experts profess that there is a strong correlation between early and deeply ingrained patterns of gender identity and adult sexual orientation. Others believe that it's a matter of genetics. Another biological theory holds that homosexuality is caused by hormonal imbalance. Professionals recognize homosexuality as a different style of sexual preference. In 1973, the American Psychiatric Association declared that homosexuality could not be classified as a mental disorder and concluded that there is no major difference in psychological adjustment between homosexuals and heterosexuals. There are no findings that distinguish one group from the other based on mental health or hormonal balance. Sexual orientation seems to be formed from a constellation of inconsistent and inconclusive factors. No one knows why, in a given family, one child may choose a same-sex lifestyle.

In most areas of our lives, we use our knowledge as a guide to help our children develop appropriate behavior. Sexual preference is different in that there are no rules and little knowledge. No one pattern of childrearing has emerged as an influencing factor in a child's sexual proclivity. It is important to recognize that *feeling attracted to the same sex does not constitute homosexuality.* As a girl, didn't you admire a beautiful actress or a cheerleader or a woman who seemed to really have her act together? As a boy, didn't you idealize some male figure—the coach, a school leader, or a famous athlete? You may even have had a crush on these people or dreamt about them. It may have frightened you, but it didn't cause you to choose a homosexual life-style.

IDENTITY STRUGGLES OF AN ADOLESCENT

Recently, I was invited to teach a class about relationships at a secondary school. When I arrived, I was overwhelmed by the enthusiastic welcome I received from the class counselor. He said that this was to be the day that a teenage boy was going to "come out of the closet." The young man had volunteered to reveal his darkest secret. But why, I asked apprehensively, would you encourage a young man to expose himself to a group of fellow students who were struggling with their own identity crisis? The counselor explained that such a disclosure would be a liberating experience for the boy and an extraordinary learning experience for his peers.

I asked the counselor if he realized how dangerous such a revelation could be for everyone concerned. How did he know that the 16-year-old was, in fact, a homosexual? The teen, like so many young people, may have experimented with one or two or even three same-sex encounters as part of an adolescent process to establish a sense of his sexual identity. This experimentation does not in any way lock a person into a particular life-style. Even if the person experienced good feelings, these feelings may be tied up with the excitement of engaging in a clandestine affair, in expressing one's independence by defying the accepted roles of society, or in stimulating erotic areas that have never been explored before.

The counselor explained that many students had revealed intimate secrets in the past, and the experience had served as a catharsis. Each member of the group had pledged an oath of secrecy and promised never to disclose to family or friends any of the secrets shared in this confidential encounter. Nothing, however, could convince me that such a disclosure was healthy.

The class proceeded as scheduled. The 16-year-old exposed his darkest secret. As I looked around the room, I caught one teen elbowing another in an attempt to suppress his nervous laughter. These two students were obviously not emotionally ready for such a disclosure. I wondered how many others were confused and frightened as they identified with the pudgy, acne-complected youth with the vacillating voice who was the featured celebrity of the day. He answered a barrage of personal questions. Yes, he had had a same-sex affair with two different people. Yes, he had visited a gay bar with his friends. He chose not to describe how he displayed his affection in a sexual encounter. No, he hadn't told his parents yet and he wasn't sure when he would. No, he had never approached a student at school for sex. Yes, he felt an attraction for girls, but he had had a sexual experience only with the two boys.

After the session ended, the boy remained seated. He looked drained. He had cried. He had laughed. He had become the "sexpert" for one class period. Each student thanked the young man for sharing. A few students shook his hand, but only two had the courage to embrace him. If anyone ever needed to be hugged, it was this boy.

I shudder to think about the consequences of this encounter. My sense is that if only one group member broke the oath of confidentiality, the news would become public within a matter of hours. In the course of 45 minutes, this boy had revealed a truth that could pigeonhole him for the rest of his life. Is he a homosexual? I doubt it! Is he testing the limits of his sexuality? Absolutely. Has he had enough experience to know what life-style is most appealing? Of course not! I couldn't help but wonder how his self-perception will change once his acne clears, his voice deepens, and he successfully chooses his path in life.

We would know just as little about this young man's lifelong sexual propensity if he had disclosed that his first two encounters had been heterosexual. But that experience would not have been worthy of revelation. In his search for acceptance and approval, he may have embarked on an anxiety-packed search for identity. And so you see once again that children need the sensitive support of their parents and extended family as they seek assistance in maturing to sexually healthy adults. Being "askable" may protect your child from seeking guidance from the wrong source.

Since sexuality is the dominant theme throughout the adolescent years, you can see how profoundly it shapes the personality. In offering information about homosexuality to your children, you and they may find comfort and greater understanding about this behavior from a conclusion published by Dr. Alfred Kinsey, based on years of research and interviews with hundreds of people. Dr. Kinsey concluded that every person has an individual sexual orientation that can be measured on a scale of "0" through "6." A person who is exclusively heterosexual is classified as "0." A person who is exclusively homosexual would be classified as a "6." People who have experienced a varying degree of sexual preference fall somewhere along the continuum. Using this measure, along with data collected by other researchers, it is estimated that approximately 2 percent of men and 1 percent of women are exclusively homosexual, while approximately 23 percent of men and 14 percent of women have had both homosexual and heterosexual experiences. The majority of people in the United States, however (75 percent of men and 85 percent of women), are exclusively heterosexual. Establishing one's place along the continuum allows a person to see that he or she is not locked into an either/or sexual orientation.

Because we know so little about the origin of homosexuality, parents often worry needlessly that their child will be induced into this life-style. Many parents fear that exposure to homosexuality may be dangerous to their child. Homosexuality is not contagious. However, if your child does show a clear pattern of homosexual relationships over a period of time, you must recognize that there is little you can do other than to reaffirm your love and support. The reasons for this preference are not well established, but one thing we do know is that there appears to be no choice in the matter. I have seen parents unjustly blame themselves for a biological and psychological persuasion that is not proven to be related to overprotective parenting, negligent parenting, or single parenting.

All of us have hopes and desires for our children's happiness and safety. When these plans are frustrated or abandoned, *the loving decision is to continue to love.* Parents must not feel responsible for every decision a child makes. Life is filled with many influencing factors about which we have little understanding and far less control.

People who are driven toward the gay life-style face many struggles as they swim against the tide of acceptable sexuality. Too often they lead double lives, guarding themselves from persecution. I have heard it said that perhaps homosexuality is the most genuine sexual expression. People who freely express their life-style are usually closely in touch with their ability to express their emotions. Some have gone so far as to say that a homosexual male is the essence of what manliness is all about. This man has no need for pretense. He knows who he is and acts in accordance with his needs and desires.

I struggle with my sense of authenticity when discussing homosexuality. Personally, I passionately believe in the doctrine of freedom of choice, when, of course, it is not exploitative of others. I choose my friends for qualities that I respect and value. These values do not include what a person does in the privacy of his or her own bedroom. However, when it comes to my own children, my feelings are less clear. I hope that they will form a lasting relationship with another who best complements their needs. I would be happiest if they found a partner of the opposite sex, but I would be accepting if they did not. In either event, I pray that they find happiness in life and that they will be guarded from persecution and prejudice. If my wishes seem in conflict with my general philosophy of freedom of choice, then I must confess that I, too, struggle, as do most people with my personal view. I do know for sure that my children are God's children and I will always love them unconditionally.

I'll end this chapter with a profound comment expressed by Anna, a sagacious 81-year-old great-grandmother. She had visited Key West, Florida, for the first time. As Anna sipped a drink in a local gay cafe, she commented on the handsome features of two young men at the adjoining table. The young woman who was hosting the trip to the Keys stated, "Grandma, he's gay!" A second person at the table then exclaimed, "What a waste!" Anna looked puzzled and then matter-of-factly stated, "Only if they don't make one another happy."

8

Sex Is Spoken Here

For the past 20 years, I have visited many schools to teach other parents' children about what is euphemistically referred to as "human growth and development." I usually speak to a combined class of 60 children or to an assembly of 300 students in a program designed to convey as much information as possible within a limited amount of time. In the past, however, I too often found that time constraints and administrators' caution prevented me from fully addressing the children's needs. So I changed my format. I still arrive at a school with a prearranged agenda, but now I request written, unsigned questions from every student as the price of admission. The response has been astounding.

The fifth- and sixth-grade students were desperate to know the meaning of words—the basic building blocks of communication. When I spoke about menstruation, they wanted to know the meaning of words like "clit" and "cherry." When I referred to nocturnal emission, they wanted to know the meaning of "boner" and "jerking off." These were the words they heard in the streets and saw scrawled on the bathroom walls. Children also heard words at home, on TV, and in the movies. They realized that these words were powerful tools, but nobody had ever explained what they meant. It became blatantly clear that before any discussion about sexuality could commence, it had to be preceded with a definition of terms.

It is only logical that we cannot have an understanding of a subject whose vocabulary is ambiguously defined. My personal suspicion is that when little children are reared on baby talk, they are being conditioned by their parents to accept slang or "dirty" language instead of the proper terminology to describe their body and their bodily functions.

As you assume the role of your child's primary sexuality educator, I recommend that you define the substance of the *words* your children use. The messages of such words can be confusing. For example, when I found "F-U-C-K" chalked across a sixth-grade blackboard at one school, I asked if anyone in the class could define the word. The students roared with laughter. "Honestly," I said with a whimsical smile, "lots of people define 'fuck' differently."

At hearing me say the word, the class was nearly on the floor, with arms bent across stomachs to contain their enormous mirth. I explained that in another class I taught, one boy thought that "fuck" was just a bad word you say when you are angry. Another boy said it was what two dogs do in a park. Finally, a demure little girl announced that she knew the answer. She explained that "fuck" was a term used to describe a robber holding up a liquor store. She felt certain of the definition because just the night before she had seen a movie in which a policeman had held a gun to a robber's head and said, "Don't move or I'll shoot—you fucker."

Defining "IT"

The language of sex becomes distorted because parents are either uncomfortable with approaching the vocabulary or they don't know how to define "IT" properly. Parents have said that they would like to use the scientific language for "IT," but they are unaccustomed to using words such as buttock, coitus, and vulva. As a result, they either ignore the "IT"s or admonish children for saying "IT."

I argue that it is *unhealthy* to use IT words and baby talk in referring to the body parts. A child who refers to his penis as "peepee" or her vagina as "hole" coupled with expressions of "dirty" in regard to elimination and "bad" related to self-pleasuring will naturally link shameful, negative, and childlike emotions to sex issues. Children who are unable to identify their body parts properly, saying, "He touched my meat" instead of "He touched my penis," may actually put their personal safety in jeopardy. During a rash of reported cases of child sexual abuse, it was a sad fact that children who identified their sexual anatomy in euphemistic and metaphoric terms presented testimony that the courts determined was non-definable and therefore invalid.

In a more amusing vein, a woman called me to make an appointment. She told me that she and her husband wanted to speak with me about "Herkamer." She stated that Herkamer was giving them a lot of heartache. "He used to be cooperative but now he's lost his vitality. Even first thing in the morning he's lethargic and lifeless. Herkamer never used to be like this before; perhaps his age is catching up with him." "How old is Herkamer?" I inquired. "He's fifty-four," the woman responded. "How is he related to you?" I asked. "What do you mean?" she queried. "Well," I continued, "is he your brother or your uncle or your child?" "No," she responded with a burst of laughter, "Herkamer is the name we call my husband's penis."

THE DANGER OF THE "IT" WORD

Three delightful teens, age 15, 16, and 17, come to the She Center to obtain birth control so they can "do IT" safely. The 15-year-old explains that she has done IT because she is in love, and that, besides, everyone in school is doing IT. If she didn't succumb to the trend, she would lose her fabulous young man. When I inquire about this special guy, she describes him in loving sighs: "He drives a 280ZX." "Tell me more," I encourage. "It's black," she continues. I wait for some more details. "And it has a gold stripe and spoked tires." Moments of silence. "Oh, yes," she adds. "He's really *built.*"

I invite her friends to join us and ask if someone would kindly define "IT" for me. I get inquiries from people who are afraid they have "IT" and others who have had oral sex and are afraid of getting "IT." Some claim that everyone is doing "IT," while those who are getting married want to know how to engage enjoyably in "IT." So with great seriousness, I ask, "What is 'IT'?"

The 16-year-old replies that doing "IT" means "taking you-know-what from you-know-where" (pointing to the zipper fly front of her jeans), and "touching IT or kissing IT or putting IT in your mouth." The 15-year-old looks shocked. She gazes pleadingly at her friends and questions, "That's IT?" "Of course," snaps her 16-year-old friend. "Oh, my God," exclaims the 15-year-old. "I thought IT meant putting his THING in your THING." I ask if by "THING" she means penis and vagina. She nods her head affirmatively and begins to cry.

This is a teen in love, maybe not by adult standards, but nevertheless sincerely, emotionally in love. She had done IT because everyone else, she believed, was doing IT, too. Her tears told me again that the language of love needs to be clearly understood, for, far too often, the penalty of assuming is to be deceived.

The truth is that we don't have a working vocabulary to distinguish between the language of love and the language of sex. Young people and adults, too, often mistake one for the other in the hope that a romantic encounter will affirm their masculinity or femininity, or will resolve their boredom, alienation, depression, anger, or curiosity. *The language of euphemism that surrounds sex blurs the distinction between sex and love.* It is no wonder that teens engage in the former, thinking it will create the latter, and then are devastated to learn that this is not always the case.

My encounter with these three teenagers is classic because it represents misinformation that may never have been acquired if a trusted adult had been available to dispel the myths of "IT." "IT," the word most frequently used to describe the meaningful aspect of one's life, it can mean anything—and frequently does. It took a stranger to define a word that belonged in the province of the home. These girls' parents should have been the educators. Probably they wanted to be, but they didn't have a clue about how to start.

Some parents have told me, "I never seem to be able to find the right time." If you are a parent who has not yet talked about "IT" with your child, notice everyday Golden Opportunities. Simply look through a newspaper or magazine for an article or advertisment related to sexuality, relationships, personal hygiene, or health care, and discuss it with your children during dinner. With a little imagination, almost any material can be transformed into a sexuality-related item. If it doesn't work out at first, it matters not. At least you have made a giant step in opening the lines of communication. With some practice in discussing everyday activities, you will begin to see how naturally you can interject information about more intimate subjects. We may not be able to protect our children from all the temptations put in their paths, nor can we be on top of every new slang word that takes on a provocative meaning. But one thing is certain: *Your children are going to hear about IT from somebody— wouldn't you rather that that person be you?*

Because we have grown up believing "IT" was too hot a subject to handle, we have learned to mask our communication about intimacy—both verbal and nonverbal. For example, Marcy hungers to hug and snuggle with her children, but has been programmed by her parents to be undemonstrative. Marcy watches the children while they sleep and visualizes herself joyfully embracing them during the day. She continues this technique until she feels as though she has the courage to begin to act on her desire. Marcy initiates a game of football with the children, saying, "I'll be the Dolphins and you'll be the Jets." The unspoken wish behind the statement is "I yearn to hug you. I hope this game will help me break a lifelong pattern of aloofness."

Seven-year-old Phillip scolds his mother for neglecting to buy his favorite cereal. Mother is able to decode the meaning of the admonition: Phillip feels neglected and unloved. Mother offers her apology for the oversight. She spends more time with Phillip. In an effort to help Phillip get in touch with his emotions, she asks, "How does it make you feel when I forget your favorite cereal?"

The same kind of mixed messages often find their way into the adult bedroom. He says, "I wish you'd turn off the TV." He means, "I'd like to make love to you tonight." She says, "Writing the brief for the trial tomorrow has really wiped me out." She means, "Not tonight, dear!" How many times have you incorrectly reacted to a request, thinking that you were responding correctly?

DECODING THE MESSAGES
LOVED ONES SEND US

The guide for good listening is easy. Its many elements include body language and eye contact, both of which invite another into one's private world. You remember body language. It is the way you used to communicate with your infant before your child learned word recognition. Nonverbal communication can be far more meaningful than actual words. It is the meaning, the feeling, and the emotion behind the message. It is conveyed by a *facial gesture* such as a frown or smile, *muscle tension,* like a quivering lip, ruffled brow, or relaxed jaw, and *vocalization,* like a sigh or moan. Eye contact confirms your undivided attention. Eyes are the windows of our emotions; you know people who have smiling eyes, sad eyes, or shifty eyes.

Active listening conveys attentiveness with a gentle touch, a warm smile, and an approving nod. It means acting as a mirror for the speaker, reflecting the words and beliefs that the speaker has expressed. Active listeners bring vitality, animation, and meaning to a conversation. Active listening does *not* edit, interpret, rescue, or deny the feelings expressed by the speaker.

> *Child says:* "I wish Uncle Bill would never kiss me."
> *Parents edits:* Child really means that he wishes Uncle Bill would kiss him sometimes.
> *Child says:* "I don't want to go to the party."
> *Parent interprets:* She really wants to go to the party but doesn't want me to know.
> *Child says:* "I don't know how to feel."
> *Parent rescues:* Forget it, it's not really important that she know.
> *Child says:* "Mr. — really frightens me."
> *Parent denies:* Don't be silly; he's a wonderful person.

Let's use active listening techniques to address the previous four examples. Notice how each strategy is designed to help the listener better understand the child's feelings and the meaning behind the message.

> *Child says:* "I wish Uncle Bill would never kiss me."
> *Parent replies:* "How do you feel when Uncle Bill kisses you?" (an *open-ended question*—it cannot be answered with a "Yes" or "No").
>
> *Child says:* "I don't want to go to the party."
> *Parent replies:* "Why don't you want to go to the party?"
> *Child says:* "I don't know how I feel."

Parent replies: "It sounds like you are really confused." (a *paraphrase* of the same statement, using different words to clarify the feeling), and adds, "Can you remember when you felt like this before?" (asking the child to *recall* a related experience or feeling to increase her reserve of knowledge).

Four-year-old Tommy keeps coming to Mom with the same questions about how the baby kittens are able to get milk from the mother cat's nipples. Assessing this as a Golden Opportunity, Mommy patiently explains the process, using picture books to illustrate the information. But no matter how many times Mommy tries to vary and clarify the answer, Tommy continues to ask the same question. Just when Mommy is about to lose patience with Tommy's daily inquiry, she begins to recognize a pattern. Tommy asks this question whenever Mommy is involved with the baby or busy with household tasks. Mommy decides that Tommy's goal may be to capture her attention. When Mommy provides Tommy with more hugs and private time together, the question is put to rest.

Active listening is the basis for all intimate communication and honest disclosure. Parents and children can develop this gift, which invites each into the other's thoughts. Children can use it later as young adults to forge enduring intimacy with a mate.

WHAT ARE YOUR "IT" WORDS?

Now for some soul searching: What were the words that you were afraid of or forbidden to mention? What were the words that were most often used on the street and written on the bathroom walls?

As an 11-year-old child, I remember a male friend admonishing me for allowing his dog to jump on me and slide his body against my leg. "Don't let him do that!" he warned. "Look at his dick. He's fucking you!" I had no idea what fucking meant at the time. I assumed that it was another word for excretion and that the dog was somehow using my leg as I would use toilet tissue. Needless to say, I never let a dog ride on my leg again. I also never asked my parents about the incident because I believed I had done something bad. It wasn't until I had gone to camp that next summer that I learned that f-u-c-k meant doing "IT."

As an adult, which of the so-called "IT" words that you find unacceptable for your children to use in public do you yourself use in the sanctity of your home?

Demure Nicole came off the school bus in tears. When her mother asked what had happened, Nicole explained that everyone in her first-grade class was going to be grounded from a scheduled field trip. "Why?" her mother asked. "Jackie yelled 'shit' out of the bus window. Then I yelled 'shit,' too. And so did Marcy and Stephanie and Nate. We got into a lot of trouble. The bus driver said that we are rude and that she will not take our class on the field trip." "You must be very upset," Mom acknowledged, using her best listening skills. "I am," Nicole confirmed. "How come you never get in trouble when *you* say 'shit'? You and Daddy say 'shit' all the time!"

This was the moment of reckoning. I suppose you could call this a forced Golden Opportunity.

✳ ✳ ✳While drying Nicole's tears with a tissue, Mom puts her arm around Nicole and continues to encourage Nicole to express her feelings. "Are these the tears of a very disappointed person?" Mom inquires. Nicole nods her head. "What else do these tears say?" Nicole responds, "They say that I hate the bus driver. I want to go on the trip. It's not fair; you never said that word was bad."

"You're right," Mom replies. "It isn't fair. How would you know if the 'shit' word was bad when Dad and I use it all the time? The truth is that it is not a nice word, and Daddy and I are wrong to use it. What has happened is that I have gotten into a bad habit and so did Daddy. 'Shit' is a bad word used to describe a bowel movement. While there is nothing bad about a bowel movement, we just don't talk about such a private thing in public, and certainly not with strangers we pass in a school bus." Mom smiles and gives Nicole a squeeze. "Your bus driver was right. It is rude to use the word in public.

"I'm sorry about the field trip. But now, I need your help. Dad and I are going to stop saying 'shit.' Whenever you hear us use the 'shit' word again, you can fine us five cents. I don't want to pay you a fine, so you can be sure that I'll get into the habit of saying 'shoot' instead of 'shit' as quickly as possible!

Because the vocabulary used to discuss sexuality is so laden with hidden meanings, often the same words that express love can express hate and disappointment. "I hate your fuckin' guts!" one film gangster snarls at the other. A different scenario is a person in tears being comforted by a friend. "I'm so fuckin' disappointed. Life has no meaning." And yet another scene may come to mind of impassioned lovers: "I need you, I love you. I want to fuck you, baby."

Usually when children experiment with the language, they are simply trying to get a better understanding of what these words mean. Often their language is shocking, and they use it at the most inappropriate times. The best way to help children use appropriate language is to become the child's living dictionary. Try not to be shocked when a child uses street language. By calmly repeating the word out loud, you can defuse its shock value and then explain to the child exactly what the word means and how it may be perceived by others when used publicly.

Mom and Dad invite five-year-old Sarah and nine-year-old Myles to join their cooking club for dinner. Just as the duck is being served, Sarah breaks into song and Myles picks up on the harmony, "Oh, Lula had a chicken, Lula had a duck, she put them on the table to see if they could fuck . . ." Mom blanches, nearly dropping the platter of duck on Sarah's head. Dad blushes, half smiles, and attempts to attract the children's attention by articulating strange sounds as though he has a bone caught in his throat. The guests smile and then laugh. Myles and Sarah repeat the verse again with a little more gusto. Dad sternly says, "That will be all. We've heard all we care to hear." Mom adds, "We'll talk about this later. But for now, I want you to stop." During dinner the children exchange mischievous glances while the guests become absorbed in discussing the culinary delights before them.

After dinner, Dad escorts the children to their room. Their timing was poor, but nonetheless, Sarah and Myles have created a Golden Opportunity.

✳ ✳ ✳Dad opens the discussion, "You kids are really good singers!" to which all three roar with laughter. "Listen, guys, I know the song is funny. But you can't sing songs like that in front of others, and I'd really prefer that you not use the 'fuck' word at all. I know you hear big people say 'fuck.' And you hear the word 'fuck' in the movies and probably on the playground. But it is not a word that Mom and I use, although we could if we wanted to. 'Fuck' is just one of those words that has many different meanings. Some people say it to be funny; some use it when they are angry or happy or confused. There are a whole bunch of good words that you can use instead, like 'darn it!' or 'shoot!'

"Actually, the real meaning of 'fuck' has nothing to do with any of these things. 'Fuck' is really a bad word or street talk for two people making love with one another. You know, when Mom and I close our door so we can have privacy to have intercourse—well, that's really what 'fuck' means." Dad kisses the children. "Hey, guys, I'd like to spend more time talking, but I must return to our company. Tomorrow Mom can answer any questions you may have and I'll help out when I get home from work. Together, we can think of other good words to use instead of 'fuck.' Besides, tonight I did all the talking. Tomorrow is your turn. I'd really like to hear your feelings about what happened tonight."

Dad handled the situation like a pro. His good humor and empathy (putting himself in the children's shoes) turned the potentially distressful experience into an everyday learning opportunity. He repeated the word often enough so that it was no longer an exposed live wire. He clearly communicated his attitude about the use of the word. He defined the word as best as he could in a brief amount of time. If more explanation is needed, Dad has assured the children that both Mom and he are askable. He stimulated their imagination to uncover appropriate words to use as alternatives. Most important, he left the doors of communication open.

Some of these words make us feel very uneasy. Even saying them in order to educate our children may be a difficult task. Try silently saying the word that causes you the most discomfort. Now do this with other words that you find equally obnoxious, like "fat," "ugly," "guts," "sleazy." Your list will be individualized because the lesson here is that what offends one may not offend another. It is fun to leaf through the dictionary and see which perfectly innocuous words sound obscene. Your vocal tone and facial expression can color any word "dirty."

You'll soon see that all words are really neutral; it's the value we impose upon them that makes them obscene. Now, while alone and looking in the mirror, say aloud all of those "dirty" words that you have found to be so difficult. Most parents who try this express how amazed they are at the ease with which they finally approached the unapproachable.

Perhaps this would be an appropriate time to give some thought to the beautiful words that describe the most intimate aspect of life. If I asked ten different people to define an intimate relationship, they would have ten different responses. How would you define:

- Love
- Friendship
- Integrity
- Honesty

- Ethics
- Trust
- Loyalty
- Caring

Make a few informal notes as you respond to each quality. This may help you stay on track in what you want to communicate to your children. Feel free to include additional qualities of an intimate relationship, such as spirituality, fairness, or empathy. As you replace the words of vulgarity with words of dignity, you become an initiator of a postive sexual communication.

PORNOGRAPHY: OBSCENITY IS IN
THE EYE OF THE BEHOLDER

As the parent group convenes, Judy exclaims, "I just learned from a
neighbor that my 12-year-old son Bobby has uncovered, in our
home, some pornographic material that I thought my husband had
kept out of sight. I had assumed that it couldn't fall into our
children's hands, but my son and his friends were playing in our
home and found the material, some of which has since been discovered in the homes of some of our neighbors. I'm furious at my
husband, even though it really isn't his fault. It's just so embarrassing!"

"Which part of it is embarrassing . . . and for whom?" I
asked. "I guess I'm the one who is most embarrassed," she replies.
"Knowing that my son and his friends as well as their parents are
aware that we read such—you know—*unsavory* material." "I think
the answer is simple," I said. "I think you ought to pack your things
and move. There's only one place for you and your family now, and
that's permanent exile! I can see the headlines now: 'Upper middle
class family banished from their community when a children's sub-
committee on pornography discovers questionable reading material
stashed in the family's home!' Are you ready to move?" I ask.

By now we have both begun to laugh. The laughter helps her
to get a better grip on the reality of the situation.

"About the anger," I continue, "I probably would feel angry
also, but not at my husband. I would feel upset at my son and his
friends. After all, there should be some code of privacy that's
maintained within your home. Your son has the right to believe that
you would respect his privacy; you have the same rights that he has.
This is a perfect time to talk about the boundaries for privacy that
you would both like to have maintained.

The next issue is Mom's feelings about the magazines. After
all, millions of people support such publications. Obviously, with
such a prolific circulation, there are some adults in the neighborhood
and many other law-abiding adults in society who do not find such
magazines to be offensive. Pornography is a subjective evaluation,
and the law protects any consenting adults who choose to purchase
explicit materials for their own enjoyment in their own home. So

. . . what should be the strategy here? A Golden Opportunity is in the making. If, as a parent, you find yourself in a similar situation that provokes embarrassment, anger, or frustration, do you:

- Ignore the incident and hope it will fade into oblivion?
- Punish the child for being curious and for looking at material that is so filthy and disgusting that it's only suitable for Mom and Dad?
- Put your house up for sale and move to another town?
- Use the occasion as an opportunity for sex education?

What elements are needed to turn this incident into a Golden Opportunity? Every element that applies to *any* learning experience applies here, as well. It begins with loving communication. Take away the mystery by openly revealing the facts, discuss how you each perceived the event, and observe what valuable lessons can be learned.

❋ ❋ ❋ The conversation may go like this:

Mom: "Bobby, I suppose it seems confusing to you that, on one hand, Dad and I were acting as responsible parents by keeping under lock and key materials that we chose for you not to see. On the other hand, if the materials are so 'bad,' then you must be wondering why we find enjoyment in reading them. The answer is that we simply think that this literature is OK for us but that it is not the proper way for you to learn about the varieties of ways in which adult men and women may view one another.

"There are certain things that we do as adults that are good but that appear to a child to be bad if they are poorly presented. Remember how upset you were when you saw baby Sue nursing from her mother's breast? You couldn't stop staring, and then you couldn't stop laughing out of confusion and fear. You later told us that you weren't sure if baby Sue was playing or actually eating her mommy's breast. It wasn't until we explained the wonderful process by which a mother nourishes her infant that you realized baby Sue wasn't being cruel, bad, or funny. Once we talked about it, it became clear that what you were seeing was quite natural and very beautiful.

"Some of the pictures in these magazines can be equally confusing until you fully understand the natural beauty of the body and the caring ways in which adults express their affection for one another. Even though you see all kinds of lovemaking on TV and at the movies, Dad and I feel that these magazines are just not an appropriate way to explain what many adults do behind their closed doors. Some people enjoy reading these magazines, and others find them to be bad or wrong. In fact, some of your friends' parents will probably become very angry at us even though we never intended for you, or their children, to see what we consider to be adult or X-rated literature.

"In the future, I hope you will come to me or Dad first whenever you are feeling curious or tempted to do something that you may feel is wrong or will get you into trouble. We won't get angry. We will do our best to help you get the right information, just as I'm doing now. In time, as you grow older and wiser, you too will decide what you consider to be right or wrong, but for now I ask that you trust our judgment."

Mom continues, holding a few of the magazines in her lap: "Bobby, I guess you are interested in learning more about sexuality. Sometimes parents forget how fast their children are growing up and forget to keep providing new information. What do you think about these magazines? What did your friends think? Why do you think people buy them? Did you see something special that you'd like to talk about? I have nothing planned that I have to do, so this is a great time for us to talk."

Such a conversation can easily be adapted to any real life situation and could just as easily have taken place between a daughter and a father. Bobby learned many things from this experience:

- Some things are OK for adults, but not OK for children.
- A locked door means *private, do not invade.*

- Opinions and attitudes change when a person has maturity and knowledge.
- There have been other times when information was needed and Bobby's parents were available then, too.
- Bobby has a clearer idea of what Mom and Dad do when they close their door.
- Not everyone buys or likes these magazines.
- X-rated means *for adults only.*
- Bobby should trust his parents' judgment for now. Later, he'll be wiser and older and able to decide for himself.
- Bobby can always go to his folks for help.
- Bobby's parents are *askable.*

BUYING INTO THE MEDIA MIRAGE

How would you define pornography? In discussing pornography, some people believe that some forms of advertising and the influence of music, lyrics, and media are as offensive as pornography and perhaps even potentially more dangerous in light of their pervasive nature. From the salacious words of advertising copy to the phallic design of the packaging, there are many sexual messages in our media. Consider:

- Shampoo products that not only put a shine on the hair but also attract lecherous looks from handsome admirers
- Mouthwashes that exchange morning bad breath for an afternoon male admirer
- Toothpaste guaranteed to win the heart of Roger or Patrick or Jimmy or John
- Perfumes and colognes said to incite aggressive, seductive reactions from others

Do you remember being 13 or 20 and feeling like an ugly duckling? Did you ever buy packaged promises that failed the test of reality, such as a "gold" whistle ring that turned your finger black or a bra that promised to make you lovable? Did you purchase candy guaranteed to reduce your weight or an athletic supporter that created a bulge designed to stimulate the most casual of crotch watchers?

Human nature draws us like a magnet to the secret formulas and magic potions that promise beauty and affirmation. It comes as no surprise that those who run after false promises continue to devalue themselves.

DISPELLING THE MEDIA MIRAGE

Claudia is not quite nine years old. She is addicted to teen magazines. The doctor says that Claudia's obsession is related to her condition of precocious puberty. Her body is developing at a faster rate than those of the rest of her friends. She has pubic hair, and her breast development requires that she wear a training bra. The purchase of Claudia's first brassiere was not as Mom and Dad had planned. They had a vision of celebrating this event as they had celebrated other milestones, like Claudia's first step, her first pair of shoes, and her first day at kindergarten. Instead, Claudia reluctantly slunk into the lingerie shop with Mom. Her slouched posture and downcast eyes clearly indicated her self-consciousness. She refused to allow anyone in the fitting room and insisted that any one of the suggested bras would do just fine. The empathetic saleswoman and Mom knew that this was not a time for teasing or criticism. This was a painful day in Claudia's life.

Mom and Dad are sensitive to the stress that this premature development has placed upon Claudia. They continue to provide loving support and assure Claudia that soon her friends will catch up and many will surpass her growth. They are particularly concerned about Claudia's obsession with the magazines. The doctor advised that Claudia's preoccupation is her method of measuring her normality against the so-called teen prototype. When Mom found a jar of breast reduction cream and bogus beauty formulas stashed away in a box, along with clipped advertisments for other magical growth retardant potions, she knew it was time to intervene. The question was how to expose these fraudulent products without appearing to ridicule or belittle Claudia's concerns. A critical view of the magazines might be interpreted as a personal attack. Once Claudia was put on the defensive, there would be no way to initiate a productive dialogue. Mom decided to create a Golden Opportunity:

✳ ✳ ✳When Claudia arrives home from school, Mom cheerfully invites her to join in looking through a male muscle magazine she allegedly has received as a sample through the mail. Claudia and her mom dunk cookies into their milk and giggle as they delve into the secret world of the muscle man. "God," Mom exclaims. "I never knew that real people came in these sizes!" As they turn to the advertising section, Mom points out the misleading ads. "There should be a law to protect innocent people from being tricked like this," she protests. "I should write a letter to the Food and Drug Administration and tell them about these junk pills, creams, and candy that claim to grow hair on a man's chest and increase his muscles.

Mom laughs and points to another advertisement. "Do you think that this powder will make your brothers lovable and popular if they stir it into their milk three times a day?" "Never!" Claudia bellows. They both laugh and turn the page. "Look at this rubbish!" Mom exclaims. Claudia moves closer for a better view. This company actually claims that they can make a man's penis grow larger!" Claudia giggles. "You know, honey," Mom now looks at Claudia with loving eyes, "there are no creams or pills that can change the shape of a person's body or make them happy or popular or lovable. There are no ointments or powders that can make a man's penis larger or smaller, just as there are no jellies or salves that can make a woman's breasts or nose or ears or toes larger or smaller." (Claudia now knows that Mom *knows*. Maybe Claudia wanted Mom to know all along so that she could confirm or deny the authenticity of the potions.) "This magazine makes boys think that girls are only interested in muscles. In fact, girls like boys and boys like girls who are kind, fun to be with, talented, smart, and not conceited.

"The body is a perfect package. People do not fall in love with one part of the body. They fall in love with the person who lives inside the body. Sometimes when people become adults, they may choose to make their nose smaller or alter the shape of their ears, but only a doctor can do that by a surgical operation. This magazine can make the average boy or man feel unsure of himself because he doesn't look like any of these pictures. I don't look like any of the women in the magazines I read either, but I know that no two people look alike (unless they are identical twins, and even they are different, because one twin can have a happy and loving personality and the other can be mean and grouchy).

"I know it's been hard for you, Claudia, because your beauty has emerged earlier than your friends'. Please be patient. I promise they'll soon catch up. I wish it would happen fast for your sake. It probably will begin by the time you are in Mrs. Rogers' class. In the meantime, while you are waiting for the slowpokes, you can get a head start on developing your talents. I've been wanting to suggest that you take art classes and improve your backhand by joining the tennis clinic. Also, I'd like to read with you a brochure that I received from a modeling school that has wonderful classes for girls your age. It sounds like you would be perfect for the program."

Mom and Claudia seal this poignant discussion with a long embrace and a kiss. Mom whispers into Claudia's ear, "Honey, I love you. I love you just the way you are!"

Out of advertisements' myths and the glorification of the current beauty trend emerges today's adult raised to the hollow echoes of sexuality propaganda. Soon she'll become tomorrow's bride and tomorrow's parent. Only you, her parent, have the ability to counteract the inflated claims with loving truths.

LOVE IS MEANT FOR BEAUTY QUEENS

An attractive 26-year-old bride of eight months confides in counseling that she and her husband have been unable to consummate their marriage. "It's not his fault," she defends him. "He's loving, warm, gentle, and very patient." She pauses, "It's me. I love to be held and caressed, but my body tenses and my vagina constricts whenever we attempt intercourse. I'm still a virgin," she confesses between tears.

The medical term for this sexual dysfunction is *vaginismus*. There is no known organic cause for the involuntary contractions of the vaginal muscles that prevent penile penetration. But there are an array of psychological problems that may interfere with a healthy emotional and physical sexual response.

After two weeks of counseling, we have ruled out such possible causes as a prior sexual trauma in the form of rape or incest. Nor is she a product of an orthodox religious home with rigid moral standards. She has never desired a homosexual relationship and definitely feels a strong sexual attraction for her husband. With gentleness and patience on the part of our gynecologist and pure-grit tolerance by our bride, a pelvic examination reveals a normal, healthy vagina.

Physical therapy consists of the gradual insertion of fingers or vaginal dilators of increasing size for a period of six to eight weeks. The prognosis is excellent once she is able to disclose and accept the psychological origin of her problem. At the fourth counseling session, the lean and attractive bride begins to uncover faded mental pictures from her childhood. "Since I was a child I have never gone swimming because I hate the way my body looks in a bathing suit. I was chubby and awkward and spent most of my high school years concealing pimples and struggling with excess weight. I always felt ugly even though I was considered talented and popular. My mother was always petite, attractive, and ultrafeminine. When my friends came over, they always commented on how pretty she was. I used to think my boyfriends were more attracted to her than to me.

"Mom used to read glamour magazines, exercise, and take good care of herself. We didn't talk much, but when we did, I always felt her disappointment in me. When I wanted to learn about sex and femininity, I would pore through Mom's beauty magazines. Somehow, when I read them, I felt closer and more connected with Mom. The only problem was that the more I read, the more hopeless I felt. I began to believe that no one could love an ugly duckling like me. Occasionally, Mom would teasingly call me 'ugly duckling.' She would laugh as if it were a joke, but I knew it was true."

The truth was out! Our 26-year-old bride believed all these years that love was meant for beauty queens. Whether her perceptions were correct is not really important. The important issue is that she truly believes in her ugliness and unworthiness, and the magazines bolstered those feelings. Her beliefs are so intense that they do not allow her to take satisfaction in being a sexual partner. Her quest to be someone other than herself has created a someone she hardly knows and certainly does not appreciate.

This well-dressed, attractive, professional woman presents the facade of confidence. Who would have suspected that she suffers today from the messages of yesterday? Perhaps she's a woman you work with. Perhaps she is someone you have known for years.

This story could just as easily have been about a man who has spent his adult years running from intimacy. He may be a loner or a Don Juan who loves women and then leaves them as a means of affirming his masculinity. Chances are he is an adult who, as a child, always felt unworthy of another's affection. He, like our bride, had no one in whom to confide, so he assumed that the media and the slick magazines were correct in their representation of the ideal man.

Many pretty little girls mature into guilt-ridden and angry women, afraid that their beauty and femininity are invitations to seduction. Some try to remain sexually unattractive by showing no interest in clothes or makeup, or by developing eating disorders. A person may overeat, substituting food for love. The added pounds and unattractive body image may become an effective tool for distancing oneself from the fear of, or the disgust for, a sexual encounter. On the other hand, a person who feels unworthy or defiled may withhold food as a form of self-punishment. Carried to the extreme, this person may die of nutritional as well as physical, emotional, and sexual starvation.

Without the guidance of a caring adult, a child is frequently unable to see that a slick-sounding "fact" is really shabby fiction. It has been estimated that only 20 percent of parents have accepted the challenge of turning fiction into fact. That means that 80 percent of America's children have been relying on false promises and misleading messages from the sellers of sex. We cannot prevent children from being exposed to the media, but we can help children become aware of the subliminal messages that abound.

"I CAN'T COPE WITHOUT MY SOAP": THE INFLUENCE OF TV

Of all media, television is cited as the most influential learning resource for all children. It is estimated that the average American child watches 26 hours of television every week. A recent survey of adolescents revealed that 51 percent watch TV an average of 3 hours or more on a school day. It's difficult to measure the exact degree of influence that TV has upon a child's gender identity and sexual behavior, but when I think of the thousands of dollars advertisers spend for even a few seconds of a commercial message, I have to assume that the impact is substantial. Many parents erroneously believe that the television is a viable substitute for parental sex education. They have said to me, "My kids know everything they need to know about sex from what they see on TV." The truth is that TV rarely portrays the average couple or the ideal for sensitive intimacy. The story line usually presents fantasy love scenes without complexity and conflict, and without mutual caring and responsibility. For impressionable adolescents, who often use TV as a model for sexual interacting, they will see sex portrayed as exciting and romantic without any mention made of contraception to avoid pregnancy or the risk of sexually transmitted disease. A recent Harris poll revealed that 45 percent of teens 12 to 17 years of age believed that TV portrayals of sexually transmitted diseases were accurate, and 41 percent believed that pregnancy and its consequences were also correctly depicted.

At 16, Carrie is a victim of the media mirage. Carrie overeats whenever she feels ugly, rejected, or frustrated. The more she eats, the farther she moves from her compulsive goal to be attractive and lovable. On one hand, the food nourishes her desire to feel satisfied. On the other, food perpetuates her undesirability. In her search for her identity, she has turned to the gossamer idols of the media. Have you spoken to a teen lately who has proudly proclaimed, "I can't cope without my soap"?

Carrie has arranged her school schedule precisely so that she arrives home in time to view her favorite soap opera on television. Every afternoon, she and her friends crowd around the television.

Will the male lead have an illicit affair? Does the child star know that she was born out of wedlock? How will the co-star cope with being raped by her uncle? Carrie's school offers no classes on sexuality education. She and her friends learn about sex through TV and at the movies. When her parents are at work, Carrie and her friends watch the Playboy cable channel. As an average child television viewer, Carrie has seen sexual encounters outside of marriage since before she was 14 years old.

WORDS PUT TO MUSIC

Messages become more impressed upon our memory when they are put to music. Remember as a child how much easier it was to learn when the information was adapted to a melodious refrain? Music is a subtle yet dynamic sexual educator.

Five years ago, I snapped a photo of a five- and six-year-old while they were happily singing along to the tune of "Push, Push in the Bush." At age five and six, the sexual messages of the music may have gone unheard. Now these girls are 15 and 16. They have had years of training to appreciate the sensual beat of the current music, whose titles speak for themselves:

"We Want Some Pussy"
"Tooling for Anus"
"Hung Like a Pony"
"Candy Licker"
"I Want Your Sex"
"Cum-On-Feel the Noise"
"Boom-Boom, Take Me to Your Room"
"Get It Girls"
"Pleasure Victim"

The passionate sounds of a woman enjoying an orgasm to an insistent musical beat are played over and over to millions of youthful listeners in the privacy of their homes and on public radio, as well as being depicted on music/video cassettes. It's impossible for a youth to escape the sexual line of today's music. It doesn't seem that long ago when your parents were concerned about the sexual inducements encouraged by the music of the Beatles and Elvis's rotating hips. Elvis would pale in the shadow of the raw and earthy sex symbols of the music industry today. Groups exist with bizarre names like Mega-Death, Venom, Heathen, Butt-Hole Surfers, and Meat Men. Concert performances may include nudity, near-nudity, and an array of erotic special effects like scantily clad women held captive in wire cages. Anyone is permitted to attend these concerts so long as beer is not sold.

The Parent Music Resource Committee is a political activist group organized with the intent to demand censorship. Presently, there are some record companies that do affix a warning label on their music that the lyrics may be considered too explicit for minors. The warning is provided as a courtesy and does not carry with it legal penalties for the buyer or sellers.

And so you see, the heroes of the music industry continue to challenge our sexual frame of reference, from the nudity of the flower children of the 1960s to the gender-blending of the androgynous rock stars of the 1980s. Is there an answer to the messages that today's children are receiving through these channels? Yes, there is. It rests on *the balance that comes from the home.* Don't wait for the media messages to change. They generate far too much profit for their creators to care about the perceptions of children. Personally, I deplore censorship of any nature. I believe that the final decision lies with the discretion of the parent and the deep faith in the value system by which a child is raised.

As a sidenote: In researching the titles of the current best-selling songs, I explained to a delightful, fresh-scrubbed teenager at a local record shop that I was writing a book on sexuality. When she called my office with the titles listed above, she whispered a request into the telephone, "Could you *please* get me a box of condoms?"

ALTERNATIVES FOR LOVING PARENTS

- Which source was your wellspring for sexuality learning?

    Your mother?   Your father?
    Your brother?   Your sister?

Your friends?   Your spouse?
Your school?   Magazines?
Books?   Television?
Music?

- How did the source affect your thinking?
- How has it colored your values?
- What did you need to know that remained a mystery?
- Were your sources accurate?
- Did your sources use words you understood? Did they use too much or too little scientific language? Was street language used?
- Were you embarrassed?
- Was your impression of your sexuality elevated or demeaned?
- How do you suppose your children will respond to their inventory of influences?
- As an askable parent, how will you influence their response?

When you feel ready to initiate a creative discussion with your child about sexuality, I hope you will find the suggestions here helpful.

- Bring home an album or cassette of current popular music. Listen to the lyrics with your children. What do they say? Are they catchy? Are they suggestive? Children are flattered when parents earnestly talk with them about their music. It's one of the teachable moments in which the child is the expert. It's a comfortable time to get a bead on how seriously they abide by the messages of the lyrics. You can share opinions about the singing stars who dress and act outrageously. Are they trying to make a statement about the changing sex stereotyping, or are they simply a commercial product? Reminisce about your own teen idols. How did they affect the way you dressed? Were there tears in your house over complaints that your hair was too long or too straggly, or that your attire was inappropriate? What songs did you sing?
- Purchase a current teen magazine and the adult version of a

similar periodical and compare the messages that advise you on how to be popular, physically alluring, and sexy. Compare the role models that typify a glamour queen and a macho heartthrob. Look at ads that promise love and romance if you buy the right toothpaste, cigarettes, perfume, or automobile. Don't forget humor. Laughing is required throughout this encounter as you break down stereotypes together.

- Buy and read magazines like *Oui, Playboy,* or *Playgirl* and confront the issues with your preteen child. Do the images portray a realistic encounter and a sensitive bonding of two loving human beings or do they convey exploitation? Do the pictures entice or repulse you? How do they make you feel about your own body image? Are there redeeming qualities to reading this material? Can it be a teaching tool for children, teens, parents, and lovers, and, if so, how?
- Talk about clothing styles or go shopping together. Let your child be the expert on what's currently stylish. Is the style appropriate for you or your child? Why? Do you dress to please yourself? Do you dress with your real or fantasized body image in mind? Do you dress to look current, even if the style doesn't compliment you?

I have included these simple tried and true experiences to stimulate your creativity. The most exciting challenges, however, are the Golden Opportunities that appear throughout this book. They are as candid as Allan Funt's camera and just as spontaneous. So, keep your eyes open. Next time, when you least expect it, a Golden Opportunity may pop up and say, "Here I am."

9

A Question of Love

Who is this child who sits across from me? Her youthful features and nervous smile are framed by a tousled hairdo; her wide eyes are subtly, but deliberately, highlighted with eyeliner.

She is a "good girl." She loves and respects her parents and has never been a problem to them. She's an excellent student with a well-rounded social life. She's much like the other young people who, when they first come to see me at my office, fidget with their hair and nervously bite their lips. They usually don't say the word "sex"—not at first.

I offer my hand in friendship, smile warmly, and ask, "What's happening in your life?" Her eyes brim with tears. "It's about this boy whom I've been dating for two years. We love each other. We really do! After college we want to marry each other." She adds, "My parents like him, too."

Now her story unfolds in a breathless run-on sentence. "He said he'll never force me to do anything I don't want to do and we won't break up or anything if we don't do IT, but I think I'd like to do IT with him before he leaves for college next month."

I ask if she has gone to her parents or to any other trusted adult for advice. She replies, "I'm afraid that Mom will be disappointed in me. If she tells my dad, he'll be really upset. I was going to ask my older brothers, but they'll only embarrass me and probably tell Mom. My parents have always said that I should come to them for *anything,* but this is different. There is no way I can win. If I don't tell them, they'll think I'm a sneak; if I do tell them, they'll probably kill me."

"Kill you?" I respond with exaggerated alarm. "You're right," I nod, "they probably will kill you! How do you think they'll do it?" I ask. "Do you think they'll use a gun or a knife, or will they slip poison into your food?" With this, we laugh. The tension eases and the young woman continues: "I want to do IT but I don't want to get pregnant or get a disease. I need to talk to someone, but I'm afraid to. My head keeps holding me back, but the feelings in my heart don't go away. What should I do?"

Here is a caring young woman who is asking for parental consent, medical sanction, and contraceptive protection. She and her boyfriend are contemporary teens (good teens), from traditional homes (good homes), whose choice of words to describe Mom and Dad's possible reaction can be translated as "I am afraid of losing my parents' love." These teens are feeling the need to express their natural sexual inclination. They also feel pressured to please their parents and affirm their personal moral code. This conflict can place adolescents in a guilt-ridden state of confusion.

Like so many other young people, this couple has been looking everywhere for advice:

- The schools say . . . be careful.
- Peers say . . . do it.
- Music says . . . it's so good.
- Some novels say . . . it hurts.
- Slick magazines say . . . it feels so nice.
- Religious leaders say . . . wait for marriage.
- Media ads say . . . go for it.
- Sexuality educators say . . . if you do, make sure it's "safe sex."

The world is filled with advice for young, confused teenagers. What is "safe sex," anyway? Does that merely mean not getting caught while doing IT? Or doing IT without becoming pregnant? Or not getting a sexually transmitted disease? Or doing everything except IT?

Why is she coming to me, a stranger, instead of her parents, I think. It's her parents, not I, who taught her to walk, who stayed up all night with her when she had the measles or mumps. I don't know their thoughts about premarital sex. I don't know their religious values. What I do know is that if I were her parents, I would feel cheated for being left out of this important and personal conversation.

STRESSES OF THE NEW SEXUALITY

You may have discussed with your friends the pressures that our children face today.

You may have voiced some definite conclusions: "I absolutely would not have an abortion!" or, "I don't care what anyone says, sex should be reserved for marriage!" It's easy to be sure of your values when you are talking hypothetically. "What if" is very different from "what is." Suppose your doctor advises you that the premature cessation of your menstrual cycle indicates an early menopause. She tells you that you are not ovulating, so you stop using birth control. Suppose your doctor is wrong. You find yourself pregnant at age 45. What will you do now? Suppose your son comes home from college with his girlfriend. He wants her to share his bedroom just as they do at school. What do you say? Suppose your 14-year-old daughter wants to get birth control. She is in love and wants to have intercourse with one very special person. What is your advice?

The confusion surrounding the new sexuality has created a need for a new profession. Sex therapists, counselors, and educators have become certified to guide people in the many choices they face. There is a popular perception that we "sexperts" have all the answers. We know how many sperm are to be found in the average ejaculate. We know how to help women have satisfying orgasms. We know how to avoid contracting sexually transmitted diseases. We have all the latest data on fantasies, erotica, and birth control devices.

We have the facts, but many of us still struggle with the half-truths of a sexually changing society. Linda, a dear friend whom I highly respect, counsels teenagers. Every day she is confronted by a teen who either is pregnant or is at risk for pregnancy. Linda does not approve of teenage pregnancy. She fears the consequences of early sexual encounters for teens who are not emotionally ready for such an adult experience. But if the teens choose not to heed her advice, it becomes her responsibility to see that they are protected from premature pregnancy and from sexually transmitted disease.

IS "NO" THE ANSWER?

In order to bridge the gap between her personal and professional views, Linda has adopted what Dr. Sol Gordon, renowned psychologist and sexuality counselor, calls the "double message" technique. This is also known as the "No, but" rule. It allows Linda to state firmly that, "No," she does not endorse intercourse for teens. She then discusses the possible physical effects of the teen's sexual behavior such as pregnancy, sexually transmitted disease, and other physical ills. She explains her concern about the effects of premature sexual activity on the teen's social and psychological well-being. She then concludes by saying, "You are now aware of all the aspects of having sex. It is obviously wiser for you to wait until you are more mature and less unsure of your own values. *But* if you choose not to take my advice, please practice safe sex by using condoms along with another form of birth control. Safe sex means that you do not exchange body fluids like semen, urine, feces, or blood from a sore or cut during lovemaking."

It seems quite natural that Pam, Linda's 17-year-old daughter, would come to Linda with her personal concerns. It was two years ago, Linda recalls, that she accompanied Pam to her first college interview. While in flight to Pennsylvania, Linda was mentally reviewing, with great pleasure, the magnificent way in which her baby daughter had emerged into a beautiful young woman. It was at this moment, Linda recalls, that her woman-child turned to her and inquired about the best form of birth control.

To say Linda was startled would be an understatement. In that instant, all of Linda's values, of which she felt so sure, were being tested. She recalls a hot flash that engulfed her body and a thumping heart that she swears could be heard for miles. Linda felt sad at the thought of her baby outgrowing her youth. She felt anxious about the disappointments that could ensue. She was fearful of the possible physical and emotional consequences of her daughter's first sexual encounter. On the other hand, she was proud that her daughter had come to her and joyful that Pam's first love was such a fine young man.

Linda confessed to Pam that despite all her knowledge about sexuality, she suddenly felt brain dead. Linda, like all of us who feel secure about many issues that we are not forced to confront personally, was faced with a challenge to her authenticity. "Yes, I believe that teens who have sex should use birth control," she thinks. But what do I believe about *my* teen having sex? Is she emotionally mature enough to handle this experience at seventeen years of age? Or would she be more prepared at seventeen years and three hundred and sixty days?" Linda knew that birth control was not the issue. If Pam had already decided to have sex, there was little that Linda could do other than talk with her about sharing, caring, commitment, and the responsibility of a love-sex relationship.

Like most parents, Linda should have been better prepared. After all, Pam had been dating the same boy exclusively for close to a year. Fortunately, Linda and Pam could use the hour or more of uninterrupted flight time to have an in-depth discussion.

Linda shares "love-sex" experiences as seen through the eyes of many teens whom she has counseled. "Too often," Linda explains, "the girl who has intercourse does so because she is 'in love' with a special young man. The boy, however, has intercourse because he is 'in love' with becoming sexual." Pam assures Mom that her relationship with Scott is different. They love and respect one another. They are responsibly planning their first sexual encounter.

As a mother, Linda can choose to:

- Forbid Pam and Scott to engage in intercourse
- Ask that they wait until they are more ready (or until Linda is more ready)
- Withhold information about birth control and sexually transmitted diseases to discourage their curiosity about intercourse
- Call Scott's parents and ask that they discourage Scott from pressuring Pam to have intercourse
- Insist that Scott and Pam not see one another anymore

- Explain the nuances of pregnancy and STD prevention along with lovemaking skills so that the first experience is joyful and meaningful

Linda decides to explain to *both* teens all of the sensual landmarks (erotic zones) of their bodies to help them see that there is more to lovemaking than intercourse. She will explain that there is a repertoire of techniques that many people find sexually satisfying, like kissing, holding, touching, manual stimulation, and pleasuring one another to orgasm. Mutually gratifying lovers explore all these plateaus for intimacy *before* committing themselves to sexual intercourse, which is the ultimate in closeness. Linda will bring home all the devices of birth control to show to Pam and Scott (a list of birth control devices appears in the Appendix) and will accompany Pam to the gynecologist for her first pelvic exam. She asks Pam to delay having intercourse until Pam has more fully discussed with Scott their expectations of becoming more intimate. Linda also suggests that Scott and Pam could first explore other lovemaking alternatives for sexual closeness. Then, if they feel that they are not succumbing to outside influences, especially peer pressure, they could proceed with their plans for intercourse.

Linda has found that she often must rethink and revise the values with which she was raised. Are the new rules superior to the old? We'll only know in time when our children grow into adults. We do know from reliable studies that the "good old days" were not as stable as the romantic reveries of the past suggest. People who "saved themselves" for marriage often spent their entire adult life searching for sexual fulfillment. Youngsters who subdued their natural sexual urges matured into unresponsive adults, often plagued by sexual guilt.

You and I are the children of yesterday. Are you content with yesterday's rules? Do you honestly feel that they are in synch with today's mores?

Linda could no more envision having had a conversation with her mother about her intentions to have intercourse than she could have imagined, in her youth, the impact of the computer age. Yet both are today's realities!

This chapter is for all the parents who would prefer an emotionally bumpy, but poignantly intimate, flight with their daughter or son to the option of abandoning the ship. It is also written for all the parents who have wished they could have talked to *their* parents about sex.

THE WHY, HOW, WHERE, AND WHEN OF RESPONSIBLE TEEN LOVEMAKING

Returning to my office one Thursday evening I am confronted by anxious parents accompanying their 15-year-old daughter to the Sex, Health, Education Center. Their mission is to determine whether or not their daughter is pregnant. Her period is two months late.

The parents make reference to some "good-for-nothing" boy who has taken advantage of their innocent little girl. The daughter privately confesses to the lab technician that she has been having unprotected intercourse since the age of 13.

Miracle of miracles, the urine test is negative. The daughter nervously giggles as each family member mentally erases the perception of a personal nightmare. "You've all been lucky this time," I comment. "But what about next time? Shall we take this opportunity to counsel with your daughter and have our doctor prescribe an appropriate contraceptive?" "There's not going to be a next time," Dad snaps as he herds the family out of the center.

Two weeks later, the daughter reappears at our doorstep. This time she is alone. She wants a pelvic exam, counseling, and birth control. In the privacy of a counseling room, Rosie candidly tells me of various sexual encounters. She wishes she could talk to her parents, but says that her dad is "impossible." Her mother would help Rosie get birth control, but "if Dad found out, he'd beat us both." Rosie's 18-year-old brother has been having sex for years, she knows, because "Dad brags about it to his friends and the family."

Rosie, like 81 percent of teens recently polled by *People* magazine, wishes she could talk to her parents about sex, but feels that she can't. She has learned about sex from her boyfriends and a couple of female confidantes. She doesn't want any lectures about the risks of sex. "I like sex. I just don't want to get pregnant yet."

With a life-size model of a uterus on my lap, I review the anatomy of the reproductive system with Rosie. In order to simulate a pelvic examination, I ask Rosie to clasp her hand shut as if she were making a fist. Into the channel created by her fingers, I gently insert a speculum, a small metal device used to dilate the vaginal canal so that the doctor can perform a Pap test for cancer cells and can examine the vaginal walls and the cervix, the mouth of the uterus. (See Appendix for diagram of pelvic exam.) I explain the mechanics of the tests for syphilis, gonorrhea, and pregnancy. I demonstrate the breast self-exam and help Rosie become at ease with touching her body for health screening purposes, contraceptive care, and self-pleasure. Rosie's aversion to self-touch makes her a poor candidate for any barrier contraceptive device that requires putting her fingers into her vagina, such as a diaphragm or sponge.

The counseling also includes pragmatic aspects of sexuality. Where do you have sex? Do you have an opportunity to shower in advance and urinate after sex? "No," Rosie says. They have sex whenever and wherever they can—in the car, at home when her boyfriend's parents are at work, at a drive-in theater, on the beach. It's usually fast and they are usually frightened that they will get caught. She wishes that it could be more romantic and less stressful, but nobody has offered them a legitimate alternative and neither one has enough money to go to a motel.

This delicate issue often is of concern to parents. They don't want their children to have sex in an unsafe setting, yet they feel as though they are overextending their liberalism by inviting their children to partake in sex in the safety and comfort of home. Yet, as one parent recently said, "If I have consented to my child having sex and I have assisted with the procurement of birth control, why shouldn't I provide a safe setting so that the experience is enjoyable and there is no fear or physical danger?" What is your opinion? My opinion is that if I were to err, I would err on the side of safety.

Before leaving the center, Rosie viewed video films on safe sex, breast self-exam, and date (or acquaintance) rape. Upon completion of the pelvic and breast exam and the laboratory tests, the doctor felt Rosie would face a far greater health risk as a pregnant teen than as a contracepted minor. Since she was healthy, he prescribed birth control pills. When Rosie left the center, she had with her a starter package of birth control pills, instructions and precautions associated with their use, a signed consent stating that she understood all the family planning methods (which was countersigned by a counselor affirming that every form of birth control had been thoroughly explained, including the risks and benefits of each method). In addition, Rosie had condoms, with illustrated instructions on their use to share with her partner.

It was necessary for Rosie to understand that there are an assortment of other contraceptive means, in case the pills had to be discontinued. It was also important for Rosie, although she objected, to open and unroll a condom over a model of a phallus that we use for demonstration purposes. It was explained that oral contraceptives did not constitute safe sex unless a condom was used as well, to minimize the risk of sexually transmitted disease.

It was a long evening for Rosie, but when she left she had all the information she needed to assume the responsibility of her sexuality. I also encouraged her to find other means for self-gratification. Part of the challenge in counseling teens is trying to help them see choices for achieving intimacy that do *not* include having sex. I reminded Rosie that her mother could become her most valuable resource if she chose to make her a confidante. With Rosie's permission, we might all talk together. Without Rosie's permission, everything that transpired between us would remain absolutely confidential. Rosie left the center with my business card. She would call if she needed me and would return to the center in three months to have her blood pressure checked before additional birth control pills could be prescribed.

Two days later, Rosie's irate father called the office threatening to dismantle the center in retaliation for the birth control we prescribed for his daughter. He had found and destroyed my card and the prescription, which his daughter had hidden inside her wallet. "It's because of you," the father yelled, "that kids are promiscuous!"

On her sixteenth birthday, Rosie returns to the center. The sweet sixteener learns that she is four months pregnant. She is in tears. Her father's "prophecy" has been fulfilled.

Who is really responsible for what has happened? Is "No" the answer to teens who ask about sex and birth control? When does a parent's protective love actually become an agent for harm? Left with no other recourse, Rosie, like most teenagers, resorted to the belief that "It won't happen to me. I've been lucky so far, so why won't I be lucky again?" Without the guidance of a trusted adult, teens succumb to their romantic nature, allowing themselves to be swept into living a personal fable. Often they naïvely think that they can't become pregnant the first time they have intercourse. Or they falsely believe that they are safe from pregnancy if they have intercourse during the middle of their menstrual cycle (actually *during* ovula tion). Some don't realize that they can become pregnant without intercourse, if the sperm happens to come in contact with the vagina by way of the labia minora (small lips of the vagina). Teens are wishful or magical thinkers when it comes to pregnancy: "It simply won't happen to me."

Ready or not—Rosie is 16 years old and four months pregnant. The options are not very pleasant:

- She may carry the pregnancy to term and raise the baby.
- She may carry the pregnancy to term and give the baby up for adoption.
- She may terminate the pregnancy with an abortion.

For those "babies" who keep their babies, parenthood engulfs their unfinished adolescence. Whatever decision she makes, a young girl's entire future is affected when she becomes pregnant in her teen years. She has limited job skills. Her ability to complete her education is hampered. If she marries for the sake of the pregnancy, statistics show that the marriage probably will end in divorce in five years. If she chooses not to marry, she quickly learns that motherhood is a full-time job.

Some young women join the ranks of a national phenomena, the "feminization of poverty." Locked into the poverty cycle without any marketable skills for liberation, these mothers, lonely and depressed, often become pregnant again within a year or two. Teen pregnancy brings the joyful innocence of childhood to a screeching halt. How can such a monumental mishap be avoided?

PREGNANCY PREVENTION BEGINS AT HOME

Primary prevention begins at home. It starts in the cradle. Remember, it's the way in which you encourage appropriate masculine and feminine behavior. It is expressed in the toys you buy, the books you read, the games you play, and the secrets you convey. Responsible sexual behavior springs from yesterday's lessons.

- The power and control issues associated with toilet training
- The sense of worth associated with baby's first step and each subsequent success
- The fairness doctrine associated with playing by the rules
- The empathy learned through playing house and dressing in costume
- The boundaries of closeness with an understanding of safe and unsafe touch
- The assertive communication skills associated with a working knowledge of the language of sexuality
- The expression of affection and erotic feelings associated with kissing, hugging, and tenderness displayed at home
- The acceptance of the natural curiosity and pleasure associated with viewing and touching the naked body
- The sex-role expectations associated with the ways in which boys are encouraged to "take charge" while girls are schooled for passivity

EQUAL BUT DIFFERENT:
THE DAMAGING DOUBLE STANDARD

How do you suppose the parents in the previous anecdote would have reacted if Rosie had been a 15-year-old boy? Do you think his father would have threatened to dismantle the office if his son had appeared at the Sex, Health, Education Center in quest of condoms? Upon finding the condoms in son's wallet, would he have discarded them? Or would he have proudly slapped his son's back as if to say, "That's my boy!"

There has always existed a double standard by which society

has measured a normal male's sex drive. It has been believed that males must relieve their natural and urgent desires. Therefore, good old Dad has prompted dear young son to get what he can whenever he can. Men have told me that they were raised on the belief that when women say "No," they really mean "Yes." "A real man never takes 'No' for an answer." This belief perpetuates the myth that girls have a limited sex drive and that they will become responsive in the hands of an adept male sexual partner. Since a girl's desire is so inhibited, the theory goes, it therefore becomes her role to control and set the limits of an intimate encounter: "Good girls . . . don't."

I assert that this fairy tale of a chaste Sleeping Beauty becoming sexually awakened by the ardor of a competent Prince Charming is one of the major reasons that *56 percent of teens in a recent Harris poll said that they did not use any form of birth control the first time they had intercourse.* And only one out of three sexually active girls between the ages of 15 and 19 uses any contraceptives. The first visit to a gynecologist or a family planning center usually comes after the fact—most often to test for pregnancy. This leads me to believe that the double standard is still pervasive: Girls do not plan in advance for fear of destroying the Sleeping Beauty myth and being perceived as an "easy lay."

What was your "first time" like for you? What was the "correct" age for you to have your first sexual encounter? Would you want the same for your children? If you waited until marriage, would you advise your children to do the same? Was it all that you hoped it would be? What information would have helped to ease your way? Honest and true, did you use birth control the first time *you* had sex?

Each time I present these questions at a parent sexuality seminar, the responses are very similar. The women usually tell of the romantic fantasy that preceded the first encounter and the disappointment that followed. "I kept thinking, is this all there is?" "It wasn't as the books promised—no violins, crescendos, or billows of white clouds." "All I can remember is that it hurt and I couldn't wait for it to be over." "I remember thinking it was wonderful, but not being sure if I had had an orgasm or not and sad that I wasn't able to ask anybody about it." "He said it was great. I said I was glad. But I silently wished I'd never have to do it again." Of course, there are women who do relate exciting, romantic first encounters, but they are in the minority.

One typical recollection is told by a 34-year-old mother. Nina did as her deeply religious family instructed and postponed intercourse until her wedding night. She did not remember ever masturbating, and nothing had ever entered her vagina—not a finger, a tampon, or a speculum. Between her awkwardness and his clumsiness, somehow the marriage was consummated.

Nina remembers dreading the next sexual exchange. She remembers feeling cheated and angry at her parents for "duping" her into believing this night was going to fulfill all her greatest dreams. When Nina's marriage ended in divorce, due in part to sexual dissatisfaction, she vowed that she would never deceive her daughter or her son as she had been deceived.

Nina has kept true to her promise. Always mindful of Golden Opportunities, she took her 10-year-old daughter and 13-year-old son to an "R" rated movie. She said, "They're going to see these kinds of movies anyway, so I decided that I'd rather we see their first one together."

After the movie, Nina took the children for pizza and they discussed the picture scene by scene. "When we were finished," Nina went on, "I felt secure that my children knew the difference between sex and love. The movie provided many examples of sex without love. I told them that sex is the act of intercourse. I used all the proper scientific names to explain that some people have sex for fun, for relief of tension, for pleasure, for making babies, for love or for lust, or for many other reasons. I explained that the best reason to have sex is for love. We went on to talk about the different kinds of love, like the love we feel for parents, siblings, God, friends, animals, and a person of the opposite sex. I didn't neglect to remind them that while men and women fall in and out of love, like Daddy and me, daddies and mommies always stay in love with their children. I reassured them that Dad and I intend to remain good friends, but that each of us will probably find another person to love. Boys and girls and men and women can, and often do, fall in and out of love many times in their life."

Nina said that her parents would never have approved of her

creative sex-education approach, but Nina hadn't approved of *their* sex-education approach, either. Nina is an askable parent. Her children know that she can be relied upon for straight answers to serious questions.

When the men in our parent group were asked to describe their first sexual experience, they had a different response. "It was fabulous!" "It was like I had earned my place into a special fraternal order of *real* men." "I had waited and anticipated so long that I was thrilled and relieved to have gotten it over with." "I was nervous and scared at first, but once I did it, I couldn't wait to do it again. I fantasized screwing every girl I met." "I was so proud of myself that I wanted to shout it from the rooftops." Some men did express disappointment or extreme tension over having to "perform," but this was the exception to the rule.

Men are usually mentored by fathers, brothers, and friends about the fine art of "doing it right." One parent tells a bittersweet story. When he was 13, he and his family were vacationing at a seaside resort. While he, his brother, and his father were playing ball, his nine-year-old sister approached holding what looked like a jellyfish in her hand. "Dad, look what I found!" she exclaimed. The 15-year-old brother grabbed her hand and screamed, "Drop it! Drop it! Do you want to get sick or pregnant?" "My little sister was so frightened," the parent recalled, "that she dropped it and ran to my father for comfort. Not having seen a condom before, I was as frightened as my sister to learn that 'jellyfish' were so dangerous.

"Later in the day I asked my brother about our sister's lethal discovery. My brother nearly fell on the floor in laughter. I'll never forget how he took this shiny foil wrapper from his wallet and led me into the shower. I watched with wide eyes as he masturbated until he got an erection and then opened the condom and unrolled it over his penis. I remember how impressed I was when his ejaculate spurted into the reservoir at the tip of the condom. He assured me that I would soon be able to 'cum' just like he did, and, when I did, he'd buy me my own condoms so I could 'get laid.'

"The next summer at the seashore I was hailed the champion of the coveted 'circle jerk,' when boys sit in a circle and ejaculate. I was the champ in having jerked off the fastest and propelled my ejaculate the longest distance. Two years later, my brother took me to 'Miss Lorraine,' who taught me everything I know about sex." He smiles. "It was both scary and exhilarating. It sure helped me know what to do when I met my first special lady. The only sad part of this story," he continues, "is that no one ever explained the myth of the jellyfish to my sister. I can only imagine what kind of thoughts she had about condoms! Today, when AIDS and sexually transmitted diseases are so rampant, girls and women need to know as much about condoms as men do."

I suggested that he recall the event with his sister. Either she'll say that it has long since been resolved, or she may review it, revise it, forgive it, and discard it from her sexual past.

VIRGINITY: AN OLD-FASHIONED WORD?

The latest surveys disclose that nearly one out of five 15-year-old girls admitted to sexual activity. More than one-half of all teens in the United States have had intercourse by the age of 17. The increase in premarital intercourse is mostly related to girls whose curiosity is beginning to match that of boys. As a result, virginity is no longer prized as a virtue in marriage. Marriage itself is no longer a prized status for men, who often are able to have all of their needs met outside of a commitment. And marriage is less appealing to women, who feel it may limit their options for personal growth and career opportunities.

However, the trend to devalue virginity has been abruptly reversed with the introduction of AIDS (Acquired Immune Deficiency Syndrome) and the new strains of antibiotic-resistant sexually transmitted diseases. A recent college poll revealed that virgins now are sought after as desirable dating partners. Teenagers are beginning to restyle their lovemaking with "safe sex" as their current buzzword (a more accurate catch phrase would be "safer sex"). These couples are "technical virgins" in that they engage in all aspects of lovemaking except penile/vaginal relations. Comments like "Sex is fun, but it's not worth the worry," and "It's not worth dying for," are becoming more the norm than the exception among responsible young adults. With AIDS education beginning in kindergarten, abstinence may well become the sexual ethic on which our children are raised.

TALKING ABOUT AIDS

In the area of personal health and safety, the need for self-knowledge becomes critical. AIDS demands that sexuality education begin at home. You are already providing AIDS prevention education to toddlers in reminding them to wipe their hands after eating and to wash their hands after urinating or moving their bowels. Good hygiene is basic everyday sexuality education. The tricky part of AIDS education is to safeguard your children without conveying ugly, negative messages about the joyful expression of sexuality. The secret is to look for Golden Opportunities.

✳ ✳ ✳Seven-year-old Rachel may be crying from a cut finger, but the blessing is that she has created a Golden Opportunity. As Rachel reaches to put her bleeding finger in her mouth, Dad gently says, "Oh no, honey, let Daddy wipe your finger. It's not a good idea to put your bleeding finger in your mouth. The blood has germs in it that may make you sick. That's why doctors and dentists wear rubber gloves when they care for people who are bleeding or care for people who have sores that are oozing with white or clear liquid that we call pus. Even now, as I help make your cut all better, I'm being careful that your blood doesn't get under my nails or caught in a crack or sore that I have on my skin. If it does, there may be some germs in this blood that will travel inside my body and they could make me sick. Even though I love you up to the sky, I don't want to get your blood inside of my body, so I am being very careful. You must be careful, too, if one of your friends at school or if Mommy or I or anybody that you know cuts themself or has a sore that may spread germs. OK?"

✳ ✳ ✳Maritsa and Martin, 11-year-old twins, are concerned about their emerging sexuality. Their insecurity about their body changes is often expressed in name calling like "you fag" and "you dyke." Mom and Dad call for a family pow-wow to discuss the damage of diminishing each other by calling one another disparaging names. In talking about the assets of kindness, Mom mentions that she recently read an article about two children who were cruelly criticized and were forced to leave school because they have AIDS. Dad adds that it's difficult enough for the children and family to deal with the disease, but the insult of name calling and harassment is greater than the pain of injury.

The subject then becomes focused on AIDS. The twins ask if the two children were contagious. "No," say Mom and Dad. "There are no known cases of AIDS that have been transmitted by children through their clothes or dishes or by using the same toilet seats or utensils. In fact, there are brothers and sisters who live together and eat, sleep, kiss, fight, and even sneeze and cough on one another, and the child with AIDS has not spread the disease to anyone else in the family." Mom and Dad continue, "Now that we're on the subject of AIDS, I heard you call each other the slang, nasty words for homosexuals. A dyke is a nasty word for lesbian, which means a woman who prefers the company of women as partners for lovemaking. And fag is the nasty word for a man who prefers another man as a partner for lovemaking. Because men often make love by putting their penis, when it is stiff and hard and ready to cum or ejaculate, into the other man's anus (which is called anal sex), these people are at a high risk for catching AIDS.

"Whenever a person transfers body fluid or semen into another—maybe through oral sex, when a woman sucks a man's penis, or through intercourse, when a man deposits his ejaculate or cum inside of a woman's body, there is a high risk of catching AIDS. That's why you hear so much about using rubbers or condoms when having intercourse, oral sex, or anal sex. It's a way to keep body fluids from being transferred from one person to another. Also, people who use drugs and share the same needle for

injecting the drugs into their body can spread AIDS from
one to the other."

Mom and Dad have created a forum for further discussion in
calling the pow-wow.

Golden Opportunities may be interwoven into an unrelated
discussion, as it was with the twins. It may begin with an article from a
newspaper or the retelling of a news report, as follows:

❋ ❋ ❋An 18-year-old is becoming a Don Juan. He is being
constantly pursued by beautiful young women. Mom and
Dad are proud of his popularity, but fearful of the risks
involved in promiscuous lovemaking. During dinner, Dad
produces an article that outlines the danger of STDs and
AIDS. Dad says, "I'd like to share some of the information
from this article with you." Son says, "Dad, I know all
about it." "I thought you would, but I found some of the
latest findings to be very interesting. It's about these new
strains of gonorrhea that are resistant to antibiotics and the
continued increase in the cases of herpes."

"Don't worry," son says, "I never have sex with
a girl unless I ask her first if she has ever had herpes.
And I look, too. If I see a white blister, I don't have sex.
"That's great," Dad affirms, "because while herpes won't
kill you, there is no cure for this virus, and the continued
outbreaks of those blisters can really put a damper on your
personal and sexual life. The article points out that some
women may have an STD, including herpes, high inside
their vagina on the cervix. They don't even know they are
infected, and you can't see anything on the outside . . .
That can be a worrisome risk when you're dating." Son
agrees.

"What about AIDS, son; are you practicing safe sex?"
Son says, "I'm sick of all the media hype about AIDS. It has
nothing to do with guys who are straight. And none of the
girls I date could be carriers of AIDS." Dad agrees that his
son is probably in the safety zone, but that he can't swear for

the girls his son is dating. "After all," Dad says, "what would happen if one of those beautiful young ladies slept with a super jock who just happened to be a bisexual?" Son shrugs as if to say, "So what!" Dad then goes on to explain that you must really know a potential sex partner well and for a long enough time that you can trust her sexual history.

Dad produces condoms. Son laughs. "Hey, Dad, nobody demands that I use those." Dad sternly replies that his son must practice safer sex by using condoms with a special spermicide called nonoxynol-9. He continued by showing his son an article about a new wide-mouthed condom (called a female condom or a vaginal shield) fashioned to fit inside a woman's vagina as a protective barrier during oral sex.

Dad affirms that having sex is a wonderful and joyful experience. "After all, Mom and I have been going at it strong for thirty years. But I do want you to avoid jumping into bed with lots of different women. And I do want you to use condoms so that you'll avoid the risk of body fluids such as semen, blood (including menstrual blood), urine, feces, or vaginal secretions entering your body. I don't need to tell you about the risk of sharing hypodermic needles because I know you wouldn't use drugs, but don't share a razor or any other gadgets, like a tattoo needle, that may inject another person's blood into your body. I don't mean to lecture, son, but lovemaking can be a risky as well as a fabulous business. By the way, have you tried petting and necking, or massage and mutual masturbation? They can be an incredible turn-on. And they are super alternatives to sex until you get to know your partner well enough to have intercourse."

THE TIME OF THEIR LIFE . . .
FOR HAVING SEX

What is the proper age for children to have sex? This is probably the single most-asked question by parents and children alike.

In this chapter you met Linda, the educated educator who has been challenged by Pam, her 17-year-old daughter, who asks, "Am I ready to have sex at seventeen or will I be more ready at seventeen and three hundred sixty days?" We each know teens who at 17 are empathetic, caring, and responsible. We also know adults who are 20 and 30 and 40 who are exploitative, ego-centered, and unable to maintain a trusting, intimate relationship. Which person is more ready for sex?

We eavesdropped on a family caught in the crisis of an ill-timed pregnancy. The father insisted that his daughter not contracept and not engage in intercourse. Can children be stopped from pursuing their sexual impulses once they have been aroused?

Nina, the divorced parent who saved her virginity for her wedding night, wants her children to understand that sex may be engaged in for fun, for adventure, for pleasure, for relief of sexual tension, for procreation, for affirmation of sexual identity, and for the relief of loneliness. Most of all, Nina believes that the best sex is achieved when it is engaged in for love. The question now is: Is there a dichotomy between the value Nina places on sex for herself and the values that she wants her children to consider before engaging in intercourse?

One couple you have not yet met is Elizabeth and Doug. They have been married for 16 years. They are a delightful couple who saved intercourse for marriage. During their three years of courtship, they engaged in a variety of lovemaking activities, none of which included penile-vaginal intromission. When they did have intercourse on their wedding night, they said it was all that they had hoped it would be. The years of getting to know one another's bodies had made them skilled lovers. Elizabeth and Doug view intercourse as a "spiritual and sacred commitment between two soul mates." Even now, they create periods of abstinence in their marriage to rekindle their sexual ardor. They have joined the sexuality group because their 12-year-old daughter and 14-year-old son have been posing questions about the "new morality," which seems to be in conflict with their religious views. Doug and Elizabeth intend to hold fast to their truths. Yet they want to respond to their children's concerns. They are curious to know how other group members are coping.

I often ask each parent to write an imaginary letter to their children telling them exactly how they feel about premarital sex. This letter is written from the head, as well as the heart. A pencil records what may be difficult to express aloud. This letter then becomes the script from which parents get their cues. The script is written in pencil so that it can be changed if parents become more evolved in their convictions. Doug's letter to his children opens like this:

Dearest Mary and Brandon:

Ever since you were babies, I have tried to give you as much information as possible to help you make wise decisions in areas where your good judgment is needed. When you were ready to walk to school alone, I reinforced the rules to cross on the green and advised you not to run the risk of jumping a yellow light or dashing across the street on red. I felt secure that I had prepared you to handle this responsibility when I wasn't around. My only hope was that you would remember the guidelines and that you wouldn't be influenced by the poor judgment of your friends or others who were not as well informed as you were.

Now, I'd like to talk to you about sex. It is also an issue that is related to your health and welfare. I have some values and attitudes that I have carefully examined. You may accept some of my thoughts and reject others, but I would like you to know exactly how I feel and how I wish you would value an intimate relationship with another person. I also will give you the telephone numbers and addresses of a female doctor, a male doctor, and a teen health center. I know that I would prefer to accompany you on your visits to them, but I will not be upset if you prefer to preserve your privacy. The most important thing is that you remain well and healthy.

And so the parent begins a dialogue about one of life's many sensitive areas. Parents mistakenly believe that children do not value their opinion about sex or about any other issue, for that matter. These same parents are usually pleasantly surprised to discover that their children appreciate a parent's judgment even though they may question its validity. Please remember that the more they object or question, the more they indicate that they are grappling with a personal conflict. And while a child may not always abide by your judgment, rest assured that your values and attitudes have been heard and will be recalled when the journey becomes rocky and confusing.

The question still remains: At what age do you advise your child to consider intercourse? As you can see, the answer rests upon many variables. What used to seem right a generation ago may seem out of step today. A person must be finely tuned to the rhythm of his or her sexual desires in order to find the correct timing. A young adult who has been raised as a sexually healthy child will know that sex should never be forced upon another and should never become a test of love, power, or control. These young adults have learned at an early age that sex is to be shared by people who trust one another and who are ready to accept the responsibility for contraception and the possibility of pregnancy or sexually transmitted disease. These young adults will be prepared for their sexual unfolding.

We often fear for our children's safety and question their ability to make the "correct" decisions as the bonds of control become less defined. But at some point, we each must loosen our grasp on our child's hand. Kahlil Gibran reminds us that our children are in fact not ours. We don't own or possess them. They only pass through us as they journey toward achieving their independence.

I remember my grandparents saying that little children create little problems, while big children produce big problems. This book is designed to help you see that sex education need not become a "big problem," but rather a joyful experience of closeness with your children. It is comforting to recognize that each of us has the opportunity *every day* to create a new dimension for awareness and equality. What better legacy of love can your child inherit?

10

When Loving Hurts

I would prefer not to include the hurtful side of love in this book designed for healthy adults who seek to expand their children's sexuality potential, but the overwhelming number of people who have been faced with the dark side of love and have transformed it into a positive growth experience can be an inspiration for us all, as well as provide strategies for healing and preventing such wounds.

The two incidents described here emerged from so-called "healthy" households. They represent the estimated 200,000 to 500,000 acts of sexual exploitation that are said to occur to female children from the ages of 4 to 13 in the United States each year. These figures mean that a female child stands a one-in-four chance of becoming victimized by the time she reaches 18 years of age. (These statistics are derived from the National Abortion Rights Action League, *The Facts About Rape and Incest,* 825 15th Street N.W., Washington, D.C. 20005—1978.)

Boys are not immune from victimization, but few cases of male molestation and mother-son relationships are reported to authorities. Some researchers estimate that incest (by stepparents, first cousins, siblings, step-siblings, and biological parents) occurs in 10 percent of American families. Other researchers believe that incest between brothers and sisters is the most common experience for unreported incestuous activity. These studies further show that when mutually engaged in by siblings close in age, it often carries into adult life neutral or positive memories for both, as opposed to the devastating effects of child-parent relationships.

TORN BETWEEN TWO LOVES

"How are you doing?" I asked, putting a comforting hand on the 13-year-old's slumped shoulder. "I'm coping," she responded bravely. "It's not the divorce," she continued. "I'm glad it's happened at last. I used to get knots in my stomach every time I heard Dad holler at Mom. Then my head would pound as I heard him coming to my room to complain about Mom. I would get angry at Mom for not appreciating Daddy. And then I would feel sorry for Dad . . . so sorry.

"For so long I believed I was the only one who could keep the family together. Now I feel dirty, used, empty."

Dad, a respected community religious leader, advised his daughter that their secret sexual encounter had been "willed by God." Daughter confessed that she knew that these sexual encounters could not be God's will, but she felt trapped between two loves and was afraid of losing both.

As the fighting between Mom and Dad increased, Dad's visits became more frequent and sexual. At the same time, daughter became so consumed with maintaining peace in the household that she strived to be the model child. She devoted herself to scholastic excellence. After school she assisted Mom with household tasks. At night she consoled Daddy.

Her self-imposed schedule didn't allow for socializing. Besides, Dad was strict about his daughter's choice of friends. He didn't permit her to go to parties or dances to which boys were invited. Now Dad was leaving. Daughter's fear of desertion had been realized. "Do you think that God is really punishing me for being bad?" she asked me.

This painful story was uncovered when in a moment of candor, daughter unburdened her soul to the school counselor. After weeks of her own soul-searching, the counselor convinced daughter that the secret must be brought into the open. "The showdown" was a nightmare. Mother embraced daughter with apologies and pledges of love. Dad blamed Mom, stating that she had pushed him into the relationship. Dad also said he was fulfilling his paternal obligation to teach his daughter about the tenderness of lovemaking. "After all, who is more qualified than a loving father?"

Family counseling has helped in drawing out the sins of her father, who was himself a product of childhood sexual abuse. Her mother has confessed her unconscious acceptance of the affair by suspecting, but denying, its existence, as a means of saving herself from the prescribed wifely obligations to cohabit and procreate. She also feared her husband's wrath and the public embarrassment involved in confronting the problem. "No one would have believed me," she asserted.

Mom and daughter were helped to recognize that they were not to blame. No one in an incestuous family is guilty of blame except the offender. The offender intimidates his trusting victims through his authoritative position, be it his physical strength, financial control, material rewards, intellectual manipulation, or emotional threats.

This 13-year-old victim said, "I can handle the divorce." She probably can. But how can she handle her feelings of worthlessness and the wrenching inability to trust her natural inclinations to love and be loved?

For those who secretly endure childhood abuse, the prognosis for a sexually fulfilling adult relationship will be guarded. Women talk of this hidden dragon who raises its ugly head at unpredictable moments. One woman stated that she never really thought about the incident until she recently met a shoe salesman who looked just like her sexually abusive uncle. She broke out in a sweat and recoiled as he reached for her leg to adjust the shoe. Another mother said she thought she had put the issue out of her mind, but now that her daughter is maturing, she's "suffocating her with caution." Women have spoken of their inability to release themselves to their lovers' embrace, of their reluctance to trust a man's gentleness, of their "deadened" sexual responses. These victims may develop sexual aversions, hostility toward men or women, and an adulthood marked by anger, isolation, and loneliness. Sometimes the feelings of unworthiness, guilt, and revenge are manifested in a life-style of prostitution, adultery, sexual exploitation, alcohol, drug abuse, or even suicide.

But for those fortunate enough to receive early intervention from a sensitive adult, the prognosis for healthy adult development is much more promising. In some instances, the child as a grown person can actually find compassion and forgive the perpetrator. With forgiveness often comes healing and the ability to release oneself from past pain. It's never too late. I have counseled women who at 55 years of age have confronted and exorcised the sexual dragon from their past.

Toby, a health educator, attempted for years to bury the memories of sitting and rocking on her Daddy's lap as a child. Yet there were times that she still could feel his erect penis resting against her thighs and buttocks. When she grew old enough to understand that it was her provocativeness that was causing the erection, she felt like a "prostitute." "I realized that I was pleasuring my father in return for favors, special attention, and toys." As a parent, Toby discouraged her daughter from having any bodily contact with Adam, her husband. Adam's sense of alienation became an increasing source of conflict at home. Toby was convinced that Adam was jealous of Jessica, their two-and-a-half-year-old daughter, and viewed his continued desire to touch her as an act of perversion. Toby made an appointment for herself and Adam to come for counseling.

During their visit, Toby realized that "Adam's problem" was really Toby's problem. Toby had "forgotten" about the seductive relationship she shared with her father. I explained that she wasn't to blame. Little girls can be appealing to daddies when they scamper around the house half-dressed or snuggle in Daddy's arms smelling delicious from a bath and baby powder. But it's always Daddy's responsibility to set the boundaries of propriety and not take advantage of his child's innocent desire to please, play, or seek affection.

Toby's enlightenment expanded Adam's understanding about Toby's sexual heritage and actually enhanced the trust and intimacy of their love relationship. This negative memory from Toby's past ended up becoming a Golden Opportunity for sexuality education.

✳ ✳ ✳Toby and Adam decided to teach their daughter about appropriate and inappropriate touch together. Making Adam part of the educational process reassured Toby that her husband had no designs of impropriety. Adam and Toby started their prevention education by taking turns bathing Jessica and referring by name to all her body parts. They also talked about simple body functions to prepare Jessica for understanding more complex functions as she gets older. "This is Jessica's nose for smelling. This is Jessica's vulva. This is Jessica's navel." Jessica will know that she owns it all. Toby and Adam will tell Jessica that no one, except Jessica, is to put their hands in her pants unless she gives them permission. The instructions are worded so as not to preclude Jessica's desire to touch herself. (Please see Chapter 4 for more information on touching.)

In time, Toby will tell Jessica about her experience with her Daddy when she was a child. Toby's calm, straightforward disclosure will illustrate to Jessica that sometimes adults do not do what is right. If this happens, children have the right to say "No" and to remove themselves from harm's way. Toby will find that her first-hand experience is a most valuable teaching tool.

Toby and Adam will play the "What if" game with Jessica: "What if Uncle Arthur were to put his hands in your panties?" or "What if nice old Mr. Greene wants to rock you on his lap?" Learning that Jessica can take charge by simply saying, "I don't like this game" or "I'm going to tell Mommy and Daddy that you want to play funny games" or simply, "Stop it, I don't like what you're doing!" provides a child with an assortment of responses to situations that don't feel comfortable.

SECRETS AND SURPRISES

In general, sexual abusers select the submissive, shy, lonely, or obedient child. To win the child's friendship, they may offer gifts or rewards. Often they initiate the relationship as a game, which may include tickling and giggling. Frequently, the offender will describe the sex-play as a special or private "secret" that must never be shared with anyone else. Since secretive play is usually sexually dangerous play, and children often confuse "secret" with "surprise," I suggest that both "secret" and "surprise" be added to your sexuality vocabulary list.

Explain to children that people who keep secrets may have something bad to hide. Secrets are a bad idea. Anyone who wants to play a secret game should be told that you don't keep secrets. Mommy and Daddy will never be angry if you tell them about a person who wants to play a secret game. Tell that person that you and Mommy and Daddy never keep secrets from one another.

You can explain that a surprise is something that you may not tell right away but that later when you do tell it, it will make someone happy. A surprise is a good idea, like a surprise party for Grandma or a surprise present for Daddy. One couple from our sexuality group was so concerned about the confusion of the words that they sponsored a family slogan and poster contest. The winning entry was displayed on the refrigerator door: "Surprises are fun; from secrets we run." The runner-up read: "Secrets are to be broken and surprises are to be safeguarded."

HELPING CHILDREN LEARN TO SAY "NO"

For generations, children have been told to obey adults and authority figures. In today's world, a parent's message must be to help children say "No" to any situation that makes a child feel uncomfortable: "If a man asks you to kiss him on the mouth, you may say, 'No, I don't like to do that.' If a person calls you a baby because you don't want to play a secret game, say, 'No,' and run away from that person and tell Mommy, Daddy, your teacher, or a policeperson." Saying "No" with confidence to anyone other than Mommy and Daddy and siblings takes practice, so I recommend playing the "What if" game and deciding if your child's "No" really sounds convincing. For example, "What would you say if a person offered you an apple as a treat for Halloween?" The child may ambivalently respond with a "No, thank you." The parent may challenge the child again, "Oh, come on, all your friends ate the apples I gave them. It's good. Take it!" The child may now be more forceful in responding "No." You can continue this exercise by using a mirror to show the child how she looks when she says "No!" and really means it.

Other safety precautions such as a guideline or checklist for your baby-sitter and the hiring of child-care workers through a certified agency can be beneficial. Some neighborhoods have established a Helping Hand concept in which a colorful hand is displayed in the window of a home that has been designated as a children's safety station for a particular street or area. Parents who work find this concept comforting. Nonworking parents often volunteer to learn safety strategies from the local police department, which is happy to assist in establishing a Helping Hand program for the neighborhood children.

You can see how the early sexual messages of self-esteem (I'm OK), touching (safe and unsafe), interpreting facial expressions and body language, communicating clearly ("No," "Yes"), recognizing feelings (anger, fear, comfort, joy), and correctly identifying the anatomy and its functions become vital safeguards against sexual abuse.

Do you think that little girls would be less victimized if they were socialized as boys are to be aggressive and self-reliant? Shouldn't we stop telling boys not to take "No" for an answer? Wouldn't we diminish the vulnerability of little boys to sexual abuse if we didn't demand of them, "Take it like a man and don't be a sissy"?

Isn't it time that we began to dissolve these and other sexual stereotypes that act as barriers to raising sexually healthy children? Next time there is a heavy package to be carried, how about calling upon your daughter instead of your son for help?

FALLING IN AND OUT OF LOVE

Falling in and out of love is becoming a common pattern for marriage. Most of the 12 million American children whose parents have divorced are "coping." In many families, the end to the bickering and constant harassment is a welcome occurrence. It appears that children are able to adapt to the single event of the divorce, but it is the chain of events that precede or follow the divorce that can make the coping more difficult.

When children understand that they are not to blame for their parents' divorce and are assured of their parents' love, they generally adapt well. Some parents report new levels of family bonding that occur after the divorce. Parents are often more available and receptive to their child's needs. A bright new frame of reference for caring and communicating is often achieved.

Parents used to endure a lifetime of unhappiness for the sake of the children, yet research reveals that children who are exposed to a forced, insincere relationship in which Mom and Dad attempt to disguise their resentment and anger for one another grow to adults with a distorted concept of marital love. Children sense when adults are pretending. Nonetheless, a divorce in the family challenges traditional values associated with love, marriage, and sexuality.

Erica's mother and father celebrated their thirtieth anniversary a week before Erica's wedding. The family prided themselves on never having produced a single divorce. Six months after the wedding, however, Erica and George knew their marriage was in trouble. Eight months later, baby Tim arrived. Erica gave up her job to become a full-time mother. The tension rose as George had to contend with the added financial burden. For five years, Erica endured George's verbal insults. When his bouts with alcohol and drugs led to physical abuse, Erica decided that she could no longer stay in the marriage for the sake of the family name. She felt a sense of relief in asking George to leave. Her guilt and shame came in seeking the approval of her parents.

In claiming her right to happiness, Erica had loosened the constraints of divorce for the rest of the family. In less than a year, Erica's aunt and uncle followed suit. Erica's aunt and her husband had been estranged for the past four years. They had formed a consensual agreement to engage in extramarital sex in order to ease loneliness and to fulfill their sexual needs. Once they saw that the family survived Erica's divorce, however, they decided not to sacrifice another year of their precious lives waiting for a miracle to salvage their relationship.

The children were shocked by the announcement. "What!" they exclaimed, "after twenty years of marriage you've decided to split? You can't do that. You guys are in love!" they insisted. "No," Dad responded. "We used to be in love, but we've grown out of love with each other. We've tried to make one another happy, but it just won't work." "Try again," exclaimed the nine-year-old daughter,

Stacy. "We'll promise to be good. I won't nag you for new clothes, Doug won't bug you for a car, and Steve won't mess around with drugs anymore."

"There is no way that you caused us to become divorced," Mom assured the children. "Please understand that there is no way that you can repair our marriage. We love you very much, but we no longer love one another as husband and wife. Dad will move out at the end of the week, but he will continue to visit us and spend time with you. Just because Dad and I fell out of love doesn't mean we can't be friends and continue to share the love we feel for you."

HINTS FOR A "HEALTHY" DIVORCE

Few adults achieve a lifelong, sexually exclusive, monogamous marriage. Serial polygamy—the practice of entering a series of legal monogamous relationships—is becoming a new form of marriage. While children appear to be resilient and capable of coping, there are issues of guilt, fear of abandonment, stress over financial security, and confusion about sex and intimacy that may affect their ability to adjust. It's possible, however, to work through tensions and come out better emotionally, as did Erica and her aunt and uncle.

For Erica's four-year-old son, Dad's absence was a blow. George may not have been a good husband, but having a male figure at home is particularly important for a young child, who looks to a nurturing father for his or her perception of feminine and masculine development. The self-focused nature of preschoolers caused Tim to feel that he was responsible for Dad's leaving. Guilt, plus the concern that he might drive Mom away, too, caused Tim to regress into temper tantrums, bedwetting, and clinging to Erica.

Tim's increased misbehavior may be seen as an Oedipal expression of guilt that he has driven Dad from home because of his competitive struggle with Dad for Mom's affection. Studies show that boys—especially preschool boys—seem to have a harder time adjusting to divorce than girls. I wonder if our socialization for boys to "take it like a man" and "repress your emotions" is partly responsible for this finding?

Despite the fact that studies show that four-year-olds are most inclined to be hurt by divorce (possibly because of the Oedipal issue), Tim's exposure to his father's physical and verbal abuse and to his father's alcohol and drug-related rages, probably would have put Tim at a greater risk of psychological damage in being raised with this distorted view of "normal" male behavior. Tim's prognosis for a healthy transition will be shaped by the way in which Mom adjusts.

Typically, the early months of divorce are characterized by disorganization and confusion, which usually peak after one year. By the second year, life settles down to a slower pace and most of the stress recedes. During this time, Tim continued to wish that a magic wand would return his family to a fairy tale existence, but the test of time reinforced the fact that Daddy was not going to live at home anymore.

Erica had special issues to work through, like reclaiming her parents' admiration and respect as she strove to recover from the dramatic assault to her self-esteem. In her attempt to gain their support, she was run ragged trying to be all things to all people: dutiful daughter, breadwinner, mother, surrogate father to Tim, homemaker, cook, and chauffeur.

Erica's stress predictably peaked at the end of the first year after the divorce. Her rigid schedule, financial burdens, and loneliness was evidenced by her overeating, chain-smoking, short temper, and propensity for tears. It was her divorced aunt who shared with Erica insights derived from professional counseling: "Erica, how long are you going to continue to give to others without getting anything back in return? People who constantly breathe out eventually wither and die unless they breathe in fresh, renewing air." Erica's aunt encouraged her to write a contract in which Erica set a realistic date by which to reduce commitments, become more self-centered, and initiate social and sexual contacts.

"Perhaps what I really need," Erica said, half jokingly, "is some great sex! I'd like to exchange my vibrator for a warm male body." "List this need as a priority," Erica's aunt instructed, "and make it happen within the month." Immediately Erica initiated a self-beautification plan. She dieted, exercised, cut down on smoking, and treated herself to a new hairdo and new makeup. She joined Parents Without Partners, where she met another divorcée with whom she agreed to share baby-sitting responsibilities. Erica fulfilled her second proviso to reduce her financial commitments by sharing living space and expenses with her new friend. With more free time, a reduced financial burden, and an improved self-image, Erica began to appreciate the joys of her single status. And she was surprised to see that her renewed enthusiasm was mirrored in Tim's improved behavior and more cheerful personality.

As Erica's life became more fulfilling, she found that she felt less hostility for George. Rather than resent his visits to Tim, she encouraged father and son to spend more time together, using the free time to pursue her own pleasures. She researched community events that father and son would enjoy attending and prepared picnic lunches to add an element of fun to daytime excursions. The more access George had to Tim, the happier and better adjusted Tim became to his new life-style. Erica also expanded Tim's contact with men by visiting Grandpa more often and attending male-oriented activities sponsored by Parents Without Partners. Erica is now looking into the Big Brother program and will enroll Tim into the Cub Scouts as soon as he is eligible. As a birthday gift, Tim received a subscription to a boys magazine club and was enrolled in a junior program at the natural history museum.

As for Erica's aunt's children, nine-year-old Stacy became withdrawn and melancholy as she saw that the break in the marriage was irreparable. She had outbursts of anger that she directed from one parent to the other as her loyalty vacillated between them. While she initially promised "not to nag for new clothes," she now demanded tokens of affection as proof that she was still loved. When Mom began to bring new romantic interests to the house, Stacy's obnoxious behavior became intolerable. It was at this time that Mom sought professional counseling for Stacy, which included family sessions as well.

Everyone welcomed the therapeutic intervention, especially Doug, the teenage son, who appreciated the opportunity to vent his embarrassment about his parents' new sexual interests. Fifteen-year-old Doug, like four-year-old Tim, was at a critical stage of his sexual development, which made him especially vulnerable to the emotional injury of divorce. Doug was busy dealing with his own sexual urges and the distinction between sexual propriety and exploration. Just when he needed Mom and Dad as healthy models for interpersonal relationships, they were modeling behavior that seemed inappropriate and reckless. All his life, Doug had accepted the fact that love and sex was something that parents shared only with one another. Now, however, less than a year after Mom and Dad said they had fallen out of love, each had new and varied sex partners.

Steve, the 17-year-old, was also shaken. He feared that his experimentation with drugs had caused his parents to grow impatient with parenting. He, like Doug, was ashamed and scornful of his parents' behavior. Finances also weighed heavy on Steve's mind. What would happen if there wasn't enough money to send him to college? For a brief time Steve resorted to drugs and sexual promiscuity to reduce his anxieties. Fortunately, the football coach took Steve in hand and encouraged Steve to seek an athletic scholarship and to pursue activities that enhanced his self-esteem. Once Steve got a part-time job and began to develop a sense of independence, he looked more kindly upon his parents' decision. It almost seemed that Steve welcomed the new challenges of divorce because they tested his ability to find successful solutions to problems.

Steve's strength was contagious. His openness in counseling helped Mom and Dad recognize that their sexual flings were conveying a distorted view of intimacy. They saw that this confusion could prompt the children to test their own femininity and masculinity with premature and irresponsible sexual activity. Their sexual abandon was encouraging the children to assign a lesser value to fidelity and a greater value to an adventurous sexual encounter. They also became aware that the children's feelings of insecurity and neglect could cause them to seek affection from other sources, often the wrong ones.

Mom and Dad decided to invite only special, significant friends to their homes. In addition, undivided private time was reserved for each child. Mom and Dad together attended Steve's football games and Stacy's piano recitals. Mom and Dad alternated trips with Steve to college interviews. Dad gave Doug insights about dating. Mom gave Doug pointers on how to ask a girl on a date and what kinds of lines girls least like to hear. Both parents took Stacy to buy her spring wardrobe. A pact was made never to pit one parent against the other and that if this did occur, the perpetrator would be grounded. With cooperation and sensitivity to one another's special needs, this nontraditional family managed to put their lives back in order within a period of three years.

One evening, after a family counseling session, they stopped at a restaurant for dinner. As they waited to be served, Mom produced a Golden Opportunity.

✳ ✳ ✳Mom removed a flower from the vase in the center of the table and inquired, "Isn't this a pretty flower?" Everyone agreed. Mom then plucked a petal from the blossom and asked again, "Is this still a pretty flower?" "Yes," they all affirmed. "Doesn't this flower remind you of our family?" she pursued. "We are a beautiful family, just like this flower," Mom said. "When you remove one member, we may look a little different, but we are still beautiful. In many respects we are *more* beautiful, because we have unearthed personal strengths to support one another in the absence of the one petal. In many ways we are a better, stronger, and more vibrant blossom. If this flower could talk, I bet it would have expressed its anger at me for removing a petal. It may even be afraid that it won't survive without its entire blossom. But once I put it back into water it will see that it has the resources to continue to live. Each petal will move over a little to fill in the space I created. If the flower could talk it probably would say, "I was sad and disappointed at first when I lost one petal. I love that petal, as I love every other petal on my blossom. But I'm feeling a new kind of love for each of the petals and a sense of pride now that I discovered how creative we are in remaking this blossom together."

DIVORCES OF A NONTRADITIONAL NATURE

In some instances, the circumstances are particularly oppressive, and it takes extraordinary human resources to rectify the injury.

I met Robin, the daughter of Marilyn and Russell, when she was 14 years old. After an ugly four-year court battle, the judge decided that joint custody would be in Robin's "best interest." Robin did not want to live with her father or her lesbian mother and her lover, but she had to abide by the court's decision. The court decided that Marilyn's sexual proclivity had no bearing upon her ability to be a good and caring mother to Robin. It also stated that a girl needed a same-sex role model, especially during the adolescent years.

As Robin's counselor, it was my task to be sure that she understood the full range of sexual preferences (see also the section on homosexuality in Chapter 7). Children and parents who possess different sexual preferences may have many conflicts about major ethical and moral issues, but that doesn't mean that their love for each other need be diminished.

We discussed why so many adults fall in and out of love. Robin approached puberty in a state of great sexual confusion, distrusting her urges and questioning her identity. She spoke of her fear of "catching her mother's lesbianism" and how she protected herself by distancing herself from other females. She was pulled between Russell's bitter criticism of Mom's lesbianism and Marilyn's denouncement of Dad's "rigid, ignorant machismo nature." Whenever Robin wore jeans, Dad cautioned her that she would develop into a dyke like her mother. Whenever she spoke kindly of her father, Marilyn reminded her that it was his narrowmindedness that was separating a natural mother-daughter bond.

When Robin was 16, she met 18-year-old Joseph. Their relationship affirmed her desire to pursue a heterosexual life-style. Tired of defending her parents against each other, and tired of proving her sexual inclination, Robin ran away from home. Now 22, Robin is a housewife and mother of two children. She has grown to appreciate her mother's courage in challenging sexual conformity, and she enjoys the friendship of her mother's lover. As for her father, Robin pities his prejudice, bitterness, and inability to rise above his ex-wife's rejection. Although Robin understands his well-intended but crude attempts to shield her from the social stigma of a nonconventional life-style, she is still unable to release the resentment she holds for her father for the years of denigration her mother has had to endure.

One woman asked that I include her divorce story in this book with the hope that it will save others from the pain she sustained. As a child she remembers her father transporting her, without her mother's resistance, to his new home, reachable only by airplane. She recalls her fear of not being able to survive without her mother, and the sadness of feeling unworthy of her mother's love. Hating her new residence and her abusive stepmother, she placed the blame on her biological mother, willing her mother's death in her own mind. Years later, she returned to the city in which she was born, but made no attempt to locate her mother.

As an adult, she searched for a mate to provide the unconditional love she felt her mother had not provided, but continued to be attracted to unhealthy relationships, which reaffirmed her unworthiness. She married an alcoholic and bore him children, whom he neglected. After years of misery, she sought the services of a social agency that supported her in divorcing her husband. The struggle for survival without the financial aid of a spouse was untenable. She lost her house and her car, and resorted to government subsidy. In the meanwhile, her husband entered an alcoholics treatment program, recovered, and remarried. He refused to provide child support, but offered to care for the children, since he and his new wife were childless.

Torn between her love for her children and her wish to see them secure, the mother reluctantly relinquished her children to the father, who relocated more than 1,000 miles away. Mother's pride prevented her from confessing to the children that she was unable to support them and herself. She simply said, "It will be in your best interest to live with your father and his new wife." Never did she tell them that her heart was breaking, nor that she was gripped with guilt. "Perhaps," she thought, "I am not capable of raising these beautiful children." And so she relinquished her children without any resistance.

It wasn't until she attempted suicide that a social worker helped her work through the tapestry of her life. She began to see the similarity between what had happened to her as a child and what had occurred with her own children. For the first time, she attempted to understand the circumstances that may have dictated her mother's decision to relinquish her as a child.

With the unconditional love from a counseling support group, she was encouraged to forgive the past so that she could get on with her life. With great fear, she contacted her aging mother, only to learn that history had, in fact, repeated itself. Her mother's life had been destroyed by anguish and guilt. She had resorted to alcohol to drown her sorrow. All these years she had yearned to see her daughter, but felt ashamed and unworthy.

Our friend used her unhappy life experience as a valuable lesson for her children's healthy growth and development. She wrote to her children and followed the letter with a telephone call avowing her love and explaining that her financial distress had forced her to make this decision in order to secure their future happiness. It's hard to say how many lives will be transformed by this mother's courage to use her past as a tool for enriching the future.

PLANNING A HEALTHY DIVORCE

Planning a healthy divorce entails a careful exploration of all the predictable reactions. Once the announcement has been made, uninterrupted private time must be provided for each child to express what she or he is feeling. "What's going on in your head? What are you feeling in your tummy? What are the tears saying?" Always keep in mind what lessons can be learned. This is your Golden Opportunity to refer to other small and big crises that you and your children have endured and overcome, like the time Timmy's bicycle was stolen or the day Margie's best friend moved to Cincinnati or when lightning destroyed the tree house. Reflect on how you and your child felt at the time. Did you cry? What did you think would happen? What did you do to accelerate the recovery? How do you feel about the incident now? Could you endure it if it happened again? How?

TIPS FOR SURVIVING
THE FIRE DRILLS OF LIFE

For every crisis that we have aggressively confronted, we have liberated new survival skills that can be recalled at a given time. I refer to these crises as the fire drills of life. They prepare us emotionally and physically to escape from a hypothetical burning building. The more experience we have with fire drills, the more competence we develop in escaping from harm's way. Recalling these positive resolutions through mental imagery is a psychologically tested technique that programs our brain and nervous system to behave according to our projected mental pictures. Each time we feed the brain imagined or real experiences, the image becomes indelibly impressed on the memory cells of the subconscious mind. At an appropriate time or on a similar occasion, the brain can be triggered into recalling the image and implementing the successful resolution.

In order to develop this powerful tool, which has been described by many as a magical approach for achieving success, close your eyes and quietly recreate a crisis in your life in which there was a successful resolution. The brain cannot distinguish between imagined or real experiences, so if you cannot think of a crisis with a solution that seems relevant to your present needs, you can redesign the resolution so that it satisfies your goal. Recreate the incident in every detail. Think of it as an instant photograph slowly developing and exposing delicate subtle nuances. Now, lock the photograph in your mind by firmly pinching the web of skin between the thumb and index finger of your right hand. This locks in the emotions and thoughts that accompany the wonderful feelings you had as you overcame the crisis.

Each time you need to call upon your survival resources for encouragement, press that junction on your right hand and you will recall this success. This process for planning ahead is called *neurolinguistic* or *psycho-cybernetic programming*. It works. Along with many of my clients, I have successfully used this technique for expanding my personal potential. Planning ahead can become a Golden Opportunity for children to make a list of all the resources they have for love and emotional support. Review with your child the person she or he would most like to call if Dad were out of town and Mom had to work late in the office. "Which person could you call if you needed a ride home from school? Whom would you feel most comfortable calling if you needed birth control? Which person is easier to talk with about personal problems? Whom might we invite to our next barbecue? If you needed a great big, delicious hug, who would be the best hugger?"

Ask your child if there are any other people you might add to this list as you get to know them better. "I met some nice people at Parents Without Partners. At the family picnic next week, we might meet some kids or adults whom we'd like to know better. Maybe, in time, we can add their names to our list."

A third Golden Opportunity is to plan with your children a daily schedule for private encounters. It is important to keep to the schedule, even if it is only 15 minutes a day. This is the time when you catch up with one another. It lays the groundwork for building intimacy in later life. Perhaps, if there were more of this intimacy in marriage, there would be fewer divorces. Take the phone off the hook, turn off the TV, and encounter one another with talk or in a playful activity, just as long as you have one another's undivided attention. This is a time to remind your child about what you appreciate about him or her. "I really appreciated your remembering to put the cap on the toothpaste. You did a great job of making your bed. Thanks for emptying the dishwasher."

One of the positive aspects of divorce is that each family member begins to pull his or her own weight. Children of divorce are usually more competent in performing basic household tasks and display more confidence in dealing with unpredictable events, such as a flat tire or blown fuse. Opportunities abound for building a sense of pride in a job well done. This nourishes self-esteem.

In a single-parent household, just as in a married household, Golden Opportunities exist for raising sexually healthy children. Small gestures of concern for each other's well-being affirm a child's sense of stability. Dad clips an article related to a child's school project. Dad spends the day with the children working in the garden because Mom's back is acting up again. Mom asks Dad if he needs to borrow the car, because his is being repaired. Just because Dad and Mom don't love each other as husband and wife, it doesn't mean that they must be hateful toward one another. You can fall out of love and still be friends. What's more, you can still be friends and fall in love with another person. This mature model for fair play takes us back to Randy, the little boy in Chapter 7 who was going to take home his bat and ball if everyone didn't play by his rules. In a healthy adult divorce, the team captains have established rules that are fair for all parties.

This ethic can extend to social and sexual issues, as well. Dad baby-sits for Mom because she has an important gala she must attend. Mom keeps the children on one of Dad's visitation weekends because he really wants to go skiing. If a child criticizes a parent, the other parent helps a child to see the parent's deed or action in a more objective light.

Mom and Dad can make it clear that the love they feel for the children is constant and unconditional. All decisions concerning the children will be made by both parents. The children are therefore put on guard not to play one parent against the other. One parent will likewise not pit one child against the other parent to gain affection, favors, or information about the ex-spouse. When Mom looks good, Dad will remember to compliment her in front of the children. Mom will comment when Dad gets a haircut or looks particularly sharp. These gestures of cooperation add to the child's positive sexual messages for the future.

For introspective children who have difficulty putting into words their sense of loss and need for affection, I propose two adjuncts to the healthy divorce: the purchase of a diary and the acquisition of a small animal, such as a kitten or puppy. A diary is a marvelous private way for children to write from their heart what their tongue is unable to express. I often suggest that each diary addition be closed with "I learned . . ." "I relearned . . ." "I was surprised to learn. . . ."

Writing notes to other family members often becomes a successful alternative for children to broach a subject that may be too difficult to verbalize. Writing a note also gives the recipient time to respond in a calm, rational way.

The small furry animal may not sound quite as appealing as a diary when there are so many new responsibilities that demand your attention. But the Golden Opportunities that it affords may be well worth the effort. The animal will provide for your child a new outlet for giving and receiving attention and affection. The added responsibility may distract a child from dwelling on the emptier household. Caring for another, be it a less fortunate person or a helpless animal, is a proven way to overcome depression. Aside from the warm, wonderful feel of a furry animal, there is the humor that accompanies its antics. At a painful time in a child's life there is nothing more valuable than humor.

Caring for animals, plants, and people is an everyday opportunity for sexuality education. After all, it takes tender care to give and receive the love of another.

SPECIAL CONCERNS OF CHILDREN DURING SAD TIMES

I believe that single parents, regardless of their sex, are as competent as married parents in raising sexually healthy children. I don't see that your children will have sexual concerns that differ from those of any other normal child progressing through life, except for two issues.

The first issue is: How do you explain to your child that a parent is unloving, especially if the parent is abusive or molesting? A more common example is a parent who promises to visit a child but often cancels at the last minute. A parent may ignore a child's birthday or be unavailable for phone calls and special events.

I believe, as do many progressive educators, that it is foolhardy to protect the neglectful parent. The parent is wrong in not acknowledging a birthday. To claim otherwise is to confuse the child. Loving someone requires that you do not demean them or constantly disappoint and ignore their needs. Loving a person increases that person's sense of security, trust, and self-worth. If a parent does not fulfill these requirements, then she or he is not a loving parent. Whatever the reason, this parent is an unhealthy role model who consistently brings pain to the child's life. Sadly, I have met many adults who continue to wait for a display of love from an indifferent parent, even though their parent has not acknowledged them for years.

Some adults move in and out of casual relationships looking for the love of this neglectful parent. Some marry spouses twice their age, hoping that this person will fill their longing for parental love. Some go through life distrusting people of the neglectful parent's sex or isolating themselves from heterosexual activities if the parent is of the opposite sex. Feelings of unworthiness and guilt may haunt this child-adult for all of his or her life.

It is kinder and wiser to acknowledge that the negligent parent is being unloving. It should be explained that these people can only love themselves, or more probably dislike themselves with such an intensity that they are incapable of loving another. The child should be told not to expect love from this sad person. Other sources of love should be identified, such as aunts, uncles, grandparents, siblings, and, of course, the custodial parent. The child should be assured that he or she is very lovable and that many people will appreciate and love him or her as he or she grows older: "You'll recognize the people who truly love you because they will tell you how special you are. These people will smile at you and tell you how happy they are for your successes. They will be sad for you when you feel hurt. You will be able to call them for assistance when I'm at work or just to tell them something that is important to you. These people will look forward to being with you to share special occasions, like birthdays and holidays. You are a lucky child because you have many people from whom to pick and choose. It doesn't make sense to choose a person to love if that person does not love you in return. There are plenty of others to take this unworthy person's place."

The other special issue is that of dating. Divorced parents may find that their children are critical of a single parent's need for affection. The child may be fearful that the new sexual interest will undermine his or her relationship with the parent. Some parents insist that any encounters be outside of the home. Others have baby-sitting arrangements with grandparents or trusted neighbors so that the children sleep out of the house for these special occasions. Parents can become ingenious in creating separate entrances to the sleeping quarters. One couple I know actually built a concealed wall panel that opened to one another's bedrooms from adjoining apartments. Most important to any sexual style is the consistent message to the children that they are unconditionally loved and that no thing or person will ever separate that bond.

The parent should explain to the child that everyone has a need for friends their own age. Even though the parent enjoys the time that is shared with the child, there are adult things that children do not do that the parent enjoys sharing with a friend. "We like to go to movies at night when you are sleeping. We like to go dancing and eat in fancy restaurants, just like you enjoy skipping rope and playing house or just being silly and giggly with your friends. Without friends, I would become lonely, just as you would if I didn't let you play with your friends. But I have no friend who is more important than you."

You may expand your answer to reassure a fearful child: "Although I have friends and go on dates, I always return home when the date is finished. After I date someone for a long time, I may invite you to come along with us. Sometimes after a person dates the same person for a long time and everyone in the family gets to know that person, the man and the woman may choose to get married."

You can add, if it is applicable, "I do not intend to get married for a long time, and I would not do so until everyone grew to be friends." Encourage your child to tell you what they most like or dislike about your dating. You can then address each of their concerns. The most important closure to any discussion about a new love interest is that the child will not be abandoned and that the parent's first loyalty is to the family.

MAKING LOVE WORK

Whether it is single, married, blended, or extended, every household interacts in its own unique fashion to create a special bond. Recently, I met with a group of teens to discuss the secrets of their parents' achievement in raising successful children.

It's eight o'clock on a Thursday night. I'm conducting a seminar for a group of 12- and 13-year-old students who have been recognized for their leadership skills and academic achievements. The subject is families. The question is: "What is your family's endearing quality?" Each child provides a response:

- "We always wait to eat dinner together, and each family member tells about one thing learned during the day."
- "We collect historical memorabilia and go antique hunting on weekends."
- "My folks are into health foods. We have family cooking classes. We even bake our own bread."
- "Sunday is our family day. After church we do something different each week. It's usually a surprise, like a picnic or fishing or horseback riding or visiting a relative."
- "Friday night is our family night. We light Sabbath candles, sing songs, eat a special dinner, and always invite a guest to share the evening."
- "My folks are teaching us what they call 'life skills,' like fixing a tire, planting a garden, or wiring a lamp. We even get paid for each new skill we learn."
- "My family conducts Tuesday night bingo games at a senior citizens' home, and each week one of us kids gets to help."
- "My folks sponsor a Little League team, and our family is active in sports."
- "My mom and I have a date three times a week just for us to do whatever we choose."
- "My Dad and I are taking a computer course together. Now we are programming video games."

Everyone responds, except for two students. Their silence soon draws the attention of the group. Finally, the freckle-faced, red-headed 13-year-old girl speaks: "My family's most endearing quality is that Mom and Dad finally got divorced. Now my brothers and I spend all holidays and two weekends a month with Dad and the rest of the time with Mom. It took about six months to get used to this arrangement, but now we really enjoy the time we spend together going bowling or to the movies. Sometimes it's difficult, but we don't fight anymore, and that's good."

Finally, the last child in the group responds: "Endearing?" he asks. "What can be endearing about a family whose father walks out and whose mother's only claim to fame is that she can hold her liquor better than any man in town? Sometimes I think the 'most endearing' prospect for happiness would be to close my eyes and never wake up."

The group reaches out to embrace the tearful young man. I am struck by the fact that his physical maturity, academic competence, and stoic demeanor mask the emotional pain he is enduring. I never would have guessed that this child was in desperate search of security and love. I silently thank God for providing this opportunity to help and cringe at the thought of all the cries for help that fall on deaf ears.

Fortunately, most of us will never know the tragedy of an attempted suicide by a loved one. We are lucky to have our children by our side so that we can hug them and tell them how much they are loved. It is important for young people to know that the end of one love relationship, whether it be the dissolution of a parents' marriage, the severing of a childhood romance, the relocation of a loved friend, or the death of a cherished adult, does not mean the termination of any future love.

A healthy divorce is evidence to children (and to adults) that people fall out of love and into love again when the individuals are open to new relationships. Even after the death of a loving spouse of many years, the survivor can find love and happiness in a new partner. The results of a broken teen romance may be devastating. The teen may fear that he or she will never be loved again. The depression of teens is not to be ridiculed as an expression of "puppy love." Their love is real and passionate. This is a good time to remind the child how he or she surmounted other crises. New friends, new activities, new sources of affection and recognition will go a long way toward healing a child's broken heart.

At first, sexuality may not seem at all related to suicide. But I must continue to remind you that sexuality is all of who we are.

When the boy in the teen group expressed his wish to "never wake up," he was saying, "I feel unloved. I feel unappreciated." He communicated and he was heard. Sexuality is like that. The more clearly you communicate, the more fully your needs will be met. Perhaps you have your own idea for an endearing quality that you wish to initiate in your family? What better time to begin than now?

11

The Families of
Sexually Healthy Children

I don't think that most couples would argue the fact that a successful long-term marriage is based upon the harmonious blending of one another's emotional and physical needs. This fragile ideal, however, is not easy to achieve. "Egalitarian" seems to be the buzzword that best describes this modern ideal.

At the root of this conflict is a new breed of parent whose values are grounded in a "traditional" home environment (most likely the one they had as a child) but who now seek to restructure their life-style as married adults. These parents are the product of the so-called sexual revolution.

WHAT'S SO GOOD ABOUT
THE GOOD OLD DAYS?

In the past 30 years, there have been more changes related to marriage, family life, and sexuality than there have been in the previous 200 years! And while the traditionalists decry the new family form, we have only to look to "the good old days" to be reminded of the generations of sexually repressed people who barely tapped their human potential.

Since World War II, remarkable changes have taken place within our society. The Industrial Age shifted the family from the farm to the urban community. People moved where the work was.

This forced the nuclear family to seek an extended family to substitute for the kin they had left behind.

The women's movement began to show its muscle as women became a strong force in the workplace. Women gained voting rights and sought equal rights in all areas of life. Science assisted the women's movement in the form of the birth control pill. Then, in 1973, the Supreme Court further freed women from the constraints of forced parenthood by declaring abortion to be a personal and private matter between a women and her doctor. Motherhood became a matter of choice, not chance. With increased financial security and greater sexual freedom, there is less urgency to marry and less reason to stay in an unhappy marriage, yet our desire for a trusted friendship, coupled with intimacy, love, and sex, is as strong as ever.

Although marriage may meet our basic needs for security and intimacy, the commitment is too frightening for many. Living together without a binding contract has become an appealing alternative. The concept is so common that the Bureau of the Census has created the acronym POSSLQ to designate those "Persons of the Opposite Sex Sharing Living Quarters." For women who have decided that they would be great mothers but poor marriage partners, a communal household with flexible child-care arrangements is an ideal option. A new vocabulary, such as "mended," "blended," "extended," and "open-ended" has been devised to define new family structures.

Women and men also are reexamining their desire to procreate. The financial crunch is one factor affecting their choice. Individuals are disinclined to give up a new sports car or a country retreat or a lucrative career for the pleasures of parenthood. "Later . . . maybe" is what I frequently hear, or "Not now . . . I'm not ready."

Cheryl, a 30-year-old investment banker, and her 36-year-old stockbroker husband are ready to have a child. The only problem is that they are locked into a $200,000 mortgage obligation. What should they do? Should they forfeit their home? Should Cheryl work through the pregnancy and soon after the delivery, as well? That would mean hiring a professional child-care worker to act as a surrogate parent, however, and absentee parenting doesn't approach their ideal. Whatever they decide, their solution to their economic dilemma will dictate their child's entire perspective of sexuality.

A NEW BREED OF PARENT

Meet Brett and Jeannie. Brett is the 29-year-old father of 6-month-old Marisa. While Brett's dad was a loving parent, he prided himself on never having changed a baby's diaper. In contrast, Brett attended childbirth classes with Jeannie. He coached her through eight hours of labor, vicariously sharing the pain of bearing down as baby Marisa pushed her way through the birth canal. From the moment of birth, Brett's bonding with Marisa was established. Brett now prides himself on being the only family member to bathe baby Marisa.

Jeannie is a nursing mother. Brett participates in the process, when he is home, by being present during the feedings. He uses this intimate time to communicate his love, relating the day's activities and providing Jeannie with a snack. Brett doesn't expect any rewards for participating in the parenting process. He does it because he wants to be a partner in the experience.

Jeannie and Brett have been married for two years after having tested their compatibility as roommates for a year prior to marriage. They lived together, shared expenses and household tasks, allowed each other the latitude to date others. It wasn't until they began to think about having children that they decided to tie the knot.

Jeannie was a skilled certified public accountant, but she lacked confidence in her ability to embrace the challenge of parenting. Brett promised to assist in the childrearing, but Jeannie was certain that she couldn't rely upon him any more than her mother had been able to rely upon her father. (Jeannie remembers spending no more than 15 minutes a day as a child interacting with her father.) Jeannie also knew that Brett's promising legal career depended on his ability to be available to his clients. Always the practical accountant, Jeannie saw their parenting relationship as an economic equation. Brett's earning potential surpassed hers. Therefore, Jeannie would rear the children and Brett would pursue his career.

Throughout the pregnancy, Jeannie felt ambivalent about her

decision to become a mother. She knew that she would miss the recognition, camaraderie, and income that her career offered. She worried that she would be unable to reenter the competitive job market.

Jeannie shared her concerns with no one for fear of sounding selfish, nonmaternal, or even abnormal. She brought to this pregnancy the rules for family living that she had learned from her parents. With this frame of reference, the more enthusiastically Brett planned for his shared role in parenting, the more Jeannie doubted his ability to fulfill his promises once the baby arrived.

Yet Jeannie did not want to repeat the pattern of her parents' relationship. Her mother had never complained, but Jeannie pitied her plight as a full-time wife and mother married to an overbearing workaholic who allowed her no opportunities to grow and change.

Jeannie's sisters and two brothers are in no way critical of their traditional upbringing. For them this model defined an ethical code in a society that burdens people with myriad choices. Sometimes Jeannie felt out of step in not embracing a family system that had worked for six out of seven people, including Jeannie's mother and father.

It wasn't until after Marisa's birth, during the shared intimate moments of feeding the baby, that Jeannie confessed to Brett the unfounded fears she had had about his sincerity in participating fully as a parent. Brett admitted his concern that Jeannie would mirror his memories of his mother, who always had seemed more devoted to her career and personal interests than she had to the children's welfare or to Dad's needs.

Brett's parents had chosen a relationship in which no institution, including marriage, took precedence over their "do what feels good" attitude. Since trust, intimacy, and fidelity could interfere with this approach, these were not always honored in their marriage. Brett recalls feeling insecure and expendable. Brett grew up without guidelines for sex-role modeling, since his parents chose any role that best suited their needs at the time. Without any sex-role expectations, responsibilities often remained unmet.

Brett and Jeannie have brought to their relationship many fond memories of their youth, along with some unpleasant perceptions that they chose to discard. Neither felt the need for a total overhaul, but they did have a desire for compromise in order to take for themselves the best of both life-styles.

Brett wishes that he had had more private time with his dad. Jeannie wishes that she, too, had had more time to be with her father, but remembers with greatest fondness the adventures she shared with both parents. Brett cherishes memories of intimate family gatherings to celebrate traditional holidays. From their families' models, Brett and Jeannie *created their own new parenting style.*

NEW ROLES AND RULES FOR FAMILIES

How much of your parents' behavior do you now emulate in expressing your feelings? Were your parents expressive, or did they resort to the silent treatment to avoid confrontation? Were feelings internalized or trivialized? Do you now see these behaviors as the culprits that erode intimacy in a marriage and trust in the bedroom? Can you also see how the behaviors hamper your ability to answer a child's sensitive questions candidly?

What about the display of joy and affection? You may have learned by example that affection was not to be displayed publicly. Today you may want to express your affection spontaneously, but you have been conditioned to constraint.

Which messages from home have enriched your adult relationships and which ones have you pledged to discard? When Jeannie and Brett married, they attached an addendum to their marriage vows. While this agreement is not legally binding, it has acted as a framework to define their relationship:

As we exchange our vows of love, we pledge to nourish faithfully the physical, emotional, and sexual well-being of one another. Without fear of ridicule, we will continue to introduce activities to enhance the romance and playfulness of our relationship.

Sexual infidelity will be considered an inexcusable breach of trust that will automatically compromise the covenant of our marriage contract. Birth control will be diligently practiced for six months. After that time, family planning will include no more than two children within a period of four years, with the option to renegotiate (with God's will) for one more child within the next three years.

We will share equally in assuming household tasks. Each chore will be fulfilled by the person who is most skillful or desirous to complete the task. Household tasks may be renegotiated after the birth of a baby.

All assets earned after our marriage will be jointly deposited and equally managed. All assets acquired before our marriage will be held independently. Jeannie's salary will be set aside for insurance, medical expenses, clothing, and vacations, while Brett will assume all other financial obligations. Neither of us will entertain a career offer that dictates relocating to another region of the country.

We will share major holiday celebrations with one another's families. We will maintain our traditional religious practices without demanding that either of us attend a religious service more than two times a year. We guarantee one another a minimum of one evening and one day a week for private time to be utilized without restrictions. All social engagements will be decided by mutual consent. When necessary, each of us will accommodate the other's wish to entertain business associates at least two times a month. The ballet and football will take precedence when choosing athletic activities or cultural events.

We will maintain a healthy life-style which excludes junk food and prohibits smoking in the house. We will set aside a minimum of three hours every week for exercise. Differences of opinion will be discussed as they occur. Compromises will be sought, and arguments must be resolved before bedtime and sealed with a kiss. This agreement, written in love as a nonbinding supplement to our marriage contract, may be revised as our marriage evolves and matures.

Would such an agreement help to define the roles and rules of your relationship? For Jeannie and Brett, creating the agreement provided an opportunity to analyze their parents' marriage styles, select what they themselves valued, and discard what they did not.

Brett discarded his parents' "I come first" attitude for a "Let's do things together" approach. He chose to retain his parents' spirit of adventure by planning frequent family excursions (trips to the circus or zoo) and engaging in spontaneous treks (from following animal tracks on a hike to touring local sites of interest).

Jeannie was delighted to discard the self-sacrificing maternal role, but she did choose to retain a prominent place as chief cook and half-time bottle washer. Brett exchanged a laissez-faire approach to childrearing for a code of reasonable and consistent discipline. Discarding his dad's carefree attitude, Brett opted for increased opportunities for bathing, holding, talking, and playing with Marisa.

Brett and Jeannie also rejected authoritarian rule and set up frequent family counsels instead. They made lists of activities to be shared together or pursued alone, such as museums and concerts, jogging and football, quiet game-playing and story-telling, career-enhancing opportunities, and household tasks. Jeannie produced a page from a bookkeeping ledger, which she fashioned into a monthly schedule.

Jeannie took into consideration that the schedule was constantly subject to revision for any number of reasons, from Brett's business responsibilities to Marisa's teething and sleeping patterns. If Brett had a late business appointment, Jeannie would excuse Brett from the designated morning feeding. If Jeannie had an evening Accounting Association meeting, Brett would assume all of the evening chores related to Marisa. They agreed that the person who provided Marisa's nighttime feeding would be exempt from formula-making the following morning or evening.

It would require Brett's cooperation for Jeannie to fulfill her wish to invite both their families for a monthly gathering. Brett agreed to help shop, cook, set up, and clean up, but requested that the event not conflict with a Sunday football game. He also asked that Jeannie's free half-day take place on Saturday morning or Sunday afternoon so that he could play football Saturday afternoon with his friends.

The schedule comes as close to this couple's ideal of shared parenthood as possible, with economic feasibility as the yardstick. Jeannie and Brett are creating a sexual script for their children that includes equality in decision making about the emotional, social, and financial development of the family.

With an equitable division of labor inside and outside the home, Brett may find that he is not engulfed by the pressures to be the main breadwinner. Jeannie's added source of income will reduce financial stress and allow them to relax and display joyful love for their children. Jeannie's self-sufficiency will model for Marisa confidence in asking for what she wants, be it at work, insisting on birth control, or in lovemaking. Brett's accessibility to Marisa will provide a male perspective and will increase Marisa's comfort with persons of the opposite sex. (It has even been documented that girls who have shared a nurturant relationship with their father later develop a higher degree of orgasmic satisfaction in their sexual relationships.) If Marisa were a Matthew, Mom and Dad's flexibility would shape his sensitivity and ego strength so that he would learn to be tender with women and excited by their competence and intelligence, as well.

CO-PARENTING AND SEXUAL WELL-BEING

With the availability of both parents, there are more laps to curl up in, hands to hold, and hugs to receive. (Remember, children who are raised with a nurturing touch easily recognize the dangers of unsafe touch.) Adolescents who have grown up knowing the comfort of soothing back rubs and hugs from Mom and Dad will not confuse the urgent touch of sexual need with the simple need to be held and kissed.

A son will learn not to interpret all touch as sexual. He will not fear a friendly expression of affection as a gesture of latent homosexuality.

I often think of the tearful father who spoke of the empty relationship he shared with his father. He grew up feeling like a stranger to the man he most admired. He wanted to be close to his dad, but the attempts were awkward. Neither had developed the skill to say "I love you," so they spent their adult years trying to become friends. Neither son nor father ever remembers being hugged, although they both yearned for a warm embrace. In changing the sexuality pattern for his family, this father will make sure that his children have no such remorse.

Flexible role modeling may be the giant step needed to break the double-standard cycle and to usher in a generation of men who are permitted to feel, care, and nurture, as well as women who are permitted to be assertive, competent, and self-reliant.

You can begin to see the happy potential for all the Marisas and Matthews of the next generation as they embark upon *their* career of raising sexually healthy children.

GRANDPARENTS: A MOST VALUABLE HUMAN RESOURCE

Despite the fact that many of their sexual values may be out of step with today's generation, grandparents are the senior survivors of long-term love affairs, loves lost, love rekindled, and intimacy on every level. They have much to share with youngsters who struggle with these issues. Most adults describe their rapport with grandparents as a love relationship without compare. Many have fond memories of a caring hand ruffling the hair, mending a missing button or a broken heart. The gift of selfless giving is a priceless one that our children later bring to their intimate relationships. Grandparents can be models of selfless love.

With many divorced adults attempting to raise children single-handedly, the senior generation frequently is asked to assume the role of surrogate parent. The request is becoming so common that legislators are examining new laws to safeguard personal rights and property rights of the seniors, as well as of the children. Insurance coverage for surrogate parents, especially grandparents who may be drafted into a parental role by circumstance or choice, is another emerging phenomenon. And while most grandparents love the option of baby-sitting, some speak of it as an obligation to be sandwiched between their desire for peace and quiet, their richly deserved retirement, and their loving concern for their children and grandchildren.

Doreen, a grandmother at 57, telephoned me with a problem. After raising three children, Doreen and her husband are now ready to cash in their pension and move to their retirement home, for which they have been saving for years.

Doreen confides that her conflict has to do with their oldest daughter, Brenda, who is newly divorced. For the past year, Brenda and her five-year-old son have lived with Doreen and her husband. It was the only economically feasible arrangement at the time. Recently, Brenda and her son moved out. "At long last," Doreen told me, "my husband and I thought we could have our retirement dream."

Now, however, Brenda is dating a man who is not ready for a commitment. He spends extended time with Brenda at her apartment. In order to provide private time for Brenda and to protect their grandson from the confusion of an uncommitted relationship, Doreen and her husband have become the official baby-sitters for their five-year-old grandson.

"How can we move now and jeopardize our daughter's relationship with this man? How can we risk the welfare of our grandson, who does not understand his mother's sleep-over guest? If we postpone our move, what guarantee do we have that this won't be the first of several long-term uncommitted relationships?"

Grandpa, grandma, and daughter came in for counseling. The resolution was that daughter could continue her relationship without her parents' assistance. Brenda must become a survivor.

Together we identified a network of friends who could be called upon as a surrogate family for Brenda and her son. Brenda would establish a clear code of sexual ethics that did not include sleep-over dates at home. This relationship was unfairly controlling the lives of her parents and her five-year-old son. While the separation would not be easy for any of them, Brenda and her parents were able to loosen the family ties without severing the love they felt for each other.

Brenda learned that she could survive by bartering time and services with her singles network. She didn't waste time licking her wounds when her noncommitted lover abruptly terminated the romance because Brenda was no longer available for sexual trysts. If anything, it reaffirmed her commitment to self-growth and to the welfare of her son.

Many more options for Brenda's happiness became available when she joined Parents Without Partners and accompanied her son to male-oriented activities sponsored by that organization. Brenda is creatively and assertively pulling her life together.

INTIMACY ACROSS THE MILES: GRANDPARENTS CAN BE SEX EDUCATORS, TOO

Gene and Paula regretted that their retirement retreat was located hundreds of miles from their city-bound children, although they loved the wide open spaces of "gentleperson" farming. In planning their exodus, they worked out a correspondence and visitation program with the family. They would exchange video cassettes and would augment letter writing with Sunday morning phone calls and audio cassette recordings, and visits during school vacations.

After the first six months, the family agreed that the distance actually had increased their closeness. The children were enraptured with the exciting experiences the farm had to offer. The distance diminished petty annoyances and maximized unconditional love.

It really didn't matter if the children occasionally forgot their manners or if Grandpa told the same story over again. No one wanted to mar the precious visits or telephone calls with unnecessary squabbles. The distance also encouraged creative gestures of kindness. Sending handcrafted gifts, newspaper clippings, and assorted surprises connected the families in a meaningful way.

In addition, the distance provided Golden Opportunities for sexuality education. When 11-year-old Eric returned home from one visit, he dazzled the family with a detailed report about the stud farm he had visited with his grandpa. "Wow," he exclaimed, "have you ever seen the size of a stallion's penis when he is ready to mate? It can grow in size from six or eight inches to fifteen or twenty inches! A stallion can get a mare pregnant every month that she is in heat— that's when an egg leaves her ovary. Horses are just like people that way." Eric had everyone's rapt attention as he explained that "a stud's sperm must reach the mare's egg before she can have a baby. The only difference between people and horses is that a human male has about two hundred million to five hundred million sperm in his ejaculate and a stallion has trillions of sperm! Also," Eric continued, "a human mother is pregnant for only nine months, and a mare carries her baby in her uterus for twelve months.

Grandpa hadn't missed a trick in educating Eric. For weeks Eric continued to ply the family with remembered facts and impressions. Grandpa was delighted to hear about his star pupil. "One day you'll thank me for this," Grandpa said. "This is one young man who won't be fooled about reproduction."

Eight-year-old Cheryl became an apartment-dwelling botanist after her visit to Grandma's garden club. She set up window boxes fashioned from milk containers containing seedlings from fruit pits and dried beans. She explained to her mother how plants become fertilized. "You see," she said, "when the pollen, which are like seeds, comes from the stamen of the male flower to meet the pistil of the female flower, a new flower gets born. Grandma said it was just like real people," Cheryl added. "When a daddy puts his seeds, which are really his sperm, from his penis into the mommy's vagina to meet the egg, a new flower, which is really a baby, gets born."

Grandma and Grandpa had profoundly raised the awareness of their grandchildren to the naturalness of sexuality. Mom and Dad pursued the process through visits to the zoo, aquarium, and botanical gardens.

The shrimp eggs that the family brought home from the aquarium were a continuous source of fascination as they observed the eggs hatch after being immersed in a properly prepared brine solution.

At the zoo, Eric had plenty of opportunities to comment on the sizes and shapes of the animals' anatomy. His curiosity about the parenting style of various animals, including humans, was also satisfied.

The family talked about the responsibility of parents to protect their offspring. Cheryl was reminded of the baby bird that was nested in a tree near her school. Mom suggested that Cheryl watch the fledgling as it developed its strength and its trust in its mother's advice to find the courage to fly from the nest, just as children do when they are strong and wise enough to leave their parents' side. When children go to nursery school or college, Mom said, they may be scared, but it is important for them to go so that they can grow to be independent adults.

At the botanical gardens, Cheryl parroted Grandma's profound philosophy of life. "Grandma says a new flower blossoms because of the delicate balance of the sun, water, and earth needed to make a new life. People blossom also because of the delicate balance of love and care they need to become happy and healthy."

One of the most noteworthy revelations was disclosed by 16-year-old Brian. There is no doubt that his discovery will enhance his perspective of sexuality for the rest of his life. "You know," Brian whispered in a confidential tone, "Grandma and Grandpa still do IT." Brian explained that one night when he was supposed to go to the movies with a neighbor, he returned to the farm earlier than anticipated because the theater was oversold. When he let himself into the house, he caught a glimpse of Grandma and Grandpa "making out" on the couch. He didn't know what to do, so he made himself busy in the kitchen, opening and closing the refrigerator door. "A few minutes later, when they knew I was in the house, they went upstairs and locked their door, just like you and Dad do when you're making love." He smiled and said, "It's great. I didn't know you could or would want to do IT when you get to be as old as Grandma and Grandpa."

ADOPT A GRANDPARENT

At their annual Thanksgiving evening family film festival, Louise and Dick retold the children's favorite tales about the wonderful adventures shared with their grandparents. One year, seven-year-old Bonny had a brilliant idea. "I'm sad that we never knew our grandparents, but why can't we adopt them, just like Mr. and Mrs. Gold adopted baby Jordan?"

Dick and Louise were amused at first, but eventually Bonny's suggestion seemed more appealing. "Why not?" they affirmed. The

next week, Dick, Louise, Bonny, and her brother Seth visited with a
social worker at a county convalescent home to discuss the feasibility
of "adopting" eligible grandparents. The family was offered a list of
eligible senior persons who were without any living relatives. Bonny
fell in love with a smiling, blue-eyed wheelchair-bound lady who
was a retired librarian. Seth was partial to a salty gentleman who had
had an adventurous life at sea. Both seniors were delighted with the
offer to be "adopted."

As surrogate grandparents, they would gladly share their life's
history and pass along their acquired skills and talents. In return,
Louise and Dick would include them at their family functions and
would see to it that the children visited at least twice a month. There
were no official agreements to sign, but as the relationship flour-
ished, there was no doubt that everyone had made a happy choice.

Both adopted grandparents offered Golden Opportunities for
sexuality education. You may think that guiding the elderly
woman's wheelchair and providing the assistance required by the less
able is not related to sexual health. Yet I believe that the act of doing
for another without asking for anything in return is an orgasmic
experience of a spiritual nature. The pleasure comes from the act of
giving and the knowledge that you have brought joy to another.

Associated with providing such acts is:
- The recognition that your overture is appropriate
- The ability to express your intentions clearly
- Handling the risk of rejection
- The ability to accept another's right to reject an offer of
  kindness
- The ego strength to know that a rejection is not a definition
  of self-worth

We each have our own perceived disabilities. Perhaps you perceive
yourself as being too fat, too thin, or too clumsy. Maybe you believe
that your breasts are too large or your penis is too small or your skin
is too hairy, too scaly, or too pock-marked. Less able persons raise
our consciousness of the inner beauty of humanity and the superficial
elements that too often limit a relationship. Seth and Bonny will

bring to adulthood a tenderness and unselfishness that are directly linked to the relationship shared with their adopted grandparents.

The adopted grandparents created another Golden Opportunity for sexuality education. The children grew interested in uncovering their own personal history, searching through faded photographs and contacting a genealogist to help trace their family's lineage. The family grew closer in sharing the excitement of this project. Louise created a personal birth certificate for each child, which further increased their sense of identity. The children were fascinated to learn for whom they were named and the attributes of the person whose name they now carried. Louise and Dick created countless opportunities to talk to the children about their own childhood experiences and how they compared to growing up in today's society.

OTHER BRANCHES ON THE FAMILY TREE

The concept of adopting an extended family need not be limited to grandparents. Meryl, a newly divorced mother who was overwhelmed with her adolescent daughter's sudden but constant defiance, made a financial arrangement with her social worker sister and the sister's Army sergeant husband to board her daughter for a school semester. Both daughter and mother thought that their love relationship would stand a better chance of survival if the daughter had breathing space during this turbulent time. Meryl was afraid that she was only adding to her daughter's identity confusion. After all, here were two single and sexual women who were standing on a similar threshold in life.

Both adolescent and middlescent were struggling to feel more confident about their sexuality. Both were figuring out how to be attractive and popular without being too sexual or compromising their personal values. Mom didn't want to lose her daughter to a premature love affair, and the daughter didn't want to lose her Mom to the same. While daughter was streamlining her figure, Meryl was combatting the cellulite sites.

For 20 years, Meryl had adhered to the maxim of "Good girls

don't" (and she hadn't). Now for the first time in her life, she wanted time alone to learn how to savor the pleasures of a sexual relationship.

While Meryl was sorting out her life, her daughter was benefiting from living in a two-parent household. She didn't object, as she had done at home, to making her bed and assisting with household tasks. She seemed to appreciate the structured life-style with its well-defined sex roles. In addition, she looked to the older siblings for academic and social guidance. Meryl's visits were frequent and friendly.

The hostility between single and sexual adolescent and single and sexual middlescent declined as each began to acknowledge the other's sexuality and define acceptable rules for its expression. At the end of the semester, mom and daughter resumed the loving friendship that had preceded the emotional rift.

FORGIVENESS IS THE PATH TO LOVE

Brett and Jeannie opened this chapter as a couple who had consciously chosen a new pattern of living. Their decision was made out of love without any resentment toward their parents' endeavors in raising a relatively happy family. But what of those people who have not made that transition? There are people who continue to carry hostility toward their parents and grandparents and cringe at the thought of their parents' assuming the role of their children's grandparents. I counsel many adults who face the latter dilemma.

Terri, a client of mine, confided to me that for years she carried with her resentments about her parents' authoritarian household. Now parents, Terri and her husband decided that these resentments were in conflict with their own, more democratic life-style. Rather than deprive their children of the love and affection Terri's parents wanted to give to their grandchildren, she and her husband, Peter, made a commitment to achieve family harmony.

She and Peter spent weeks rehearsing an imaginary dialogue before Terri found the courage to talk to her parents. "Our children will grow wiser from your knowledge and life experiences," she told them. "They will grow more secure from your unconditional love and kindness. They will be for you a source of pride as they share their accomplishments. When you invite their company, they will visit, if they are free. At times, and not just when we may need a baby-sitter, you can visit us, if you are free.

"Peter and I look forward to establishing a special relationship with you, but it is we who will be our children's disciplinarians. You will be their special grandparents who may spoil them with attention, not possessions. We ask that you support our decisions because you respect our judgment even though it may be in conflict with the rules that you upheld as I was growing up. Of course, when we are in your home we will respect your rules, as well. If you can live with this arrangement, we can look forward to sharing our lives together."

Terri's parents responded with a range of emotions from chagrin to defiance to disappointment to sadness. Terri and Peter had requested that they revise a lifetime of parenting behavior. Such a request is not easily granted. It took Terri's parents three weeks to answer, but when they did, they surprised her by saying that they had decided that life would be less complicated without having to make all the decisions, as they had to do in the past. They wanted to be with their grandchildren and would do their best to abide by Terri and Peter's rules.

"For the first time," Terri said, "I felt the love that comes from forgiving. I felt unburdened. I felt mature. I felt free. There was no anger, only a desire to communicate clearly and to remain in control. And what's amazing is the powerful influence it has had in helping me confront many other sensitive and even sexual issues with Peter and the children. I've learned that resolving the issues in our lives that appear unrelated to sexuality actually have a deep effect on our loving relationships in and out of the bedroom."

WHAT IS THIS THING CALLED LOVE?

In working with children to explore concepts of family, responsibility, love, and sexuality, I have fashioned an exercise that invites children to step into the shoes of their parents for just one week. During this week, they become surrogate parents of an uncooked, fragile egg, which is magically transformed into a vulnerable make-believe baby. The child assigns a gender to the egg. Facial features are drawn with felt-tip pens. Wisps of wool are added for hair. A name is chosen. Questions are raised as to which gender would be easiest to raise? What would you, as a parent, expect from a boy as opposed to a girl child? Why did you choose the name that you did for your egg child? Is your child named for someone who has special qualities that you admire? Are you going to give your egg child a religious affiliation? If so, will there be a ritual ceremony to welcome it into the fold?

A secure environment must be provided for this fragile egg child. Some children cushion or paint a milk container or decorate a shoe box with miniature nursery items. What colors do they choose for the nursery, and what types of toys do they select for a particular sex? Some children clothe their egg with status signature diapers or jeans. Subjects of safety, sustenance, health, and welfare are discussed. To leave the egg baby unattended might be interpreted as child neglect. To break the egg child would certainly be a gross form of child abuse. The economics of hiring a baby-sitter, buying food, and paying for medical expenses (especially if the egg were to crack) are explored. Sex-role expectations and parenting skills are constantly tested. The challenge of single parenting is impressively clear. Perhaps it would be easier if the parent coupled up with a neighbor or a friend to help relieve the burden of a single parent having to deal with all the responsibilities alone. The pros and cons of marriage and divorce are discussed.

What kind of love must a person have to get married? What kind of love should a person provide a spouse to keep the marriage alive? What kind of special love should a child expect? How can a parent best convey that love?

This exercise opens discussion on a wide variety of love-related issues. It certainly increases a child's respect for the role of parenting. In one short week, avenues of communication can be opened to areas of life that are too sensitive to approach directly. This Golden Opportunity can be as expansive as your imagination permits. It's fun; give it a try!

12

A Question of Answers: Putting Your New-Found Knowledge to Work

In becoming sexually evolved, you are now ready to discard attitudes that no longer harmonize with your newfound information and to hold firm to the beliefs that express your truth. Following are some questions that may help you to discard an old truth and embrace a new one:

- Are the potential rewards more appealing than maintaining the status quo?
- What will I gain?
- What will my children gain?
- How will our lives be enriched?

FOUR STEPS TO CREATING A NEW SEXUAL ENDOWMENT

In reading this book, you have already completed step one: considering some new beliefs about some old values. Step two is understanding how your sexuality is the total expression of who you are and how it shapes all your responses. The wealth of sexual information shared in these pages has enriched your understanding of the human sexual system. You also have learned ways to convey this knowledge to your children. This is the third step in bringing you closer to accepting or rejecting beliefs that have dominated your sexuality scripting since childhood.

Some people plateau at this step for some time before moving on. Significant transitions are always gradual. Don't be impatient. As you approach step four and test your newfound values, you may feel pressured by opposing emotions. You may know that the "wait until you marry" dictum of the 1950s has given way to sex and affection, but this doesn't ease your concern about your child's sexual health and emotional welfare. You may intellectually welcome the precept that sex is no longer seen as a man's need and a woman's obligation. But how can you allay your fear of a youngster's unplanned pregnancy, a broken heart, a dreaded sexually transmitted disease, or a cavalier attitude about another's emotional milestone? Yes, you believe that a person's sexual preference should be respected as a natural expression of their personality. But what of the nagging fear that your child might be influenced by some unknown factor to follow an unorthodox life-style? Of course, you know that AIDS cannot be contracted by casual contact, but what if your child chooses a playmate who has been diagnosed as having antibodies to the virus? Yes, you agree, sex is beautiful. But you may still question how you can convey its joyful qualities when precaution and protection are vital in the quest for intimacy.

These are the conflicts that tug at the heartstrings of loving, sexually enlightened parents. Is it any wonder that children are so confused when *we* continue to struggle to embrace our own sexual truths?

WHERE DO YOU STAND?

In Chapter 2 you completed a questionnaire designed to reveal your sexual beliefs. I invite you now to turn to Chapter 2 and reexamine the statements. Ask yourself:

- What conclusions can I draw from my answers?
- Are there issues about which I need more information?
- Have some of my ideas changed or become clearer as a result of reading this book?

- If necessary, can I defend my values?
- Is there any value worth defending?
- Why?
- With whom?

PUTTING YOU TO THE TEST

It is not unusual for children to ask the same sexuality question many times, repeating it at different stages of development as their world broadens and their comprehension skills expand.

Your values will be tested by the questions children ask. Are your head and heart in harmony with the message you convey? For example, suppose you have always believed that masturbation was unhealthy, but after reading this book you have decided that it is wiser for your young child to masturbate rather than sublimate this sexual energy into bed-wetting or stuttering or to express it later in life with premature sexual encounters and experimentation.

One day, your eight-year-old asks why it feels so good when she touches this special place between her legs. Intellectually, you know that information is not an invitation to obsessive behavior. Emotionally, however, you still are erasing the old tapes decreeing that masturbation is wrong. Your authenticity is being tested!

Pause to unscramble the mixed messages. Take a deep breath as you recall the answer that you have prepared for this experience. Now smile at your daughter and explain that "inside the place between your legs, called the vulva, is a special place (which feels like the tip of your nose) that is especially created to feel good when it is touched or rubbed. All girls and women have this special place, which is called the clitoris. Boys and men don't have a clitoris, only girls and women.

"Since the clitoris is a private part of your body, you should touch it only in private places such as your bedroom or in the bathroom. Private parts of the body shouldn't be touched in public places, like at school or in front of family and friends."

Despite your inner trepidation, you have easy access to the response that best describes your values. You have anticipated that such a question would arise anywhere between the ages of two-and-a-half to four years. Once the basic question is answered, you will take your cues from your daughter. You are prepared with additional information about the analogous anatomy of the penis and the clitoris if daughter pursues the subject. You may choose to draw the vulva, vagina, clitoris, urethra, and anus to better explain these important anatomical landmarks. You are also prepared to help your daughter see the hidden parts of her anatomy by showing her how to view herself with a hand-held mirror.

Daughter may ask to see mother's clitoris, which Mom may choose to keep private or may feel comfortable in exposing. Daughter may ask to touch mother's clitoris, to which mother will respond that she permits no one else to touch her clitoris, except Daddy or Dr. Smith. Mother speaks and acts in ways that harmonize with her new values concerning masturbation.

QUESTIONS, PLEASE! GUIDELINES FOR ANSWERING CHILDREN'S INQUIRIES

Questions asked by a child need to be answered in a fashion appropriate to the child's cognitive skills and emotional development, as well in consistence with a parent's sexual beliefs. Consider the range of options available in responding to a preschool child's inquiry of "Why is her tummy big?"

- You may ignore the question. (The child may soon recognize that you are nonaskable.)
- You may defer the answer until a more appropriate time. (The child may lose interest in the inquiry.)
- Your answer may be cryptic: "Because she's pregnant." (The child may be further confused in not knowing the definition of *pregnant.*)
- The answer may be simple and quick: "Because she's having a baby." (The child may feel confused and frustrated with a answer that didn't really satisfy the inquiry.)

In addition:

- Your definition may be framed by a moral view: "Pregnancy occurs when a *married man* and a *married woman* have intercourse," or "Pregnancy occurs when two people who have a special feeling for one another have intercourse in hopes of having a baby."
- The definition of intercourse for the purpose of getting pregnant may be simply defined as "when a man places his penis inside a woman's vagina and a white liquid called semen comes from the penis into the vagina. This semen contains sperm, which swim into the woman's uterus in her tummy to meet an egg. If the egg and sperm 'like' each other and join together, the woman becomes pregnant."

Your explanation may include the emotional aspects of lovemaking: "When a woman and a man love each other very much, they may want to create a baby together. The man and woman 'make love' by kissing and cuddling close together without any clothes on. When their bodies are very close to one another, the man's penis can gently be guided inside the woman's vagina. The man's penis then releases a special white fluid that is called semen."

Since children are literal in interpreting information, it is important to augment explanations with drawings, dolls, and models. Using crayons or colored marking pens to illustrate how one sperm from millions of sperm deposited in a woman's vagina swims through the uterus into the tubes (fallopian) to meet one or two ripe eggs (fraternal twins) can be understood by a child as an exciting adventure. Illustrating the uterus as the place where the baby grows becomes important to a child who may imagine a baby in a mommy's tummy surrounded by bits of chewed-up food.

Children from three to eight are usually mystified about how the penis gets into the vagina and how the baby finally exits through the same opening. Here again, drawings, dolls, and models clarify how the vagina and the uterus accommodate lovemaking, pregnancy, and childbirth. By making a loose fist, you can create a barrel-like opening to demonstrate how two fingers (like a penis) stretch and enter the opening (the vagina) and how this opening stretches nine months later to allow a baby to pass out of the uterus and become a newborn person.

You can anticipate that children from age four to eight will have many questions about pregnancy and birth. Their desire to play doctor is a signal that they are seeking answers. Most children ask if they can make babies, too. Your answer may be, "Sure, one day when you have grown to be twelve or fifteen, your body can produce the sperm/the eggs to make babies. But it's best to wait until you're married to have babies. Becoming a loving parent is a grown-up job for a mommy and daddy who love each other." You can bring to the discussion the fact that even mommies and daddies who love one another may not choose to be parents. They may make love without letting the man's sperm from his semen meet the woman's egg. It's never too early to talk about safe sex. Making love without intercourse or making love with a condom are concepts that the Surgeon General recommends be shared with children by the third grade.

Predictably, your child will ask if you make love. This is your Golden Opportunity to talk about the private caring and sharing that occur between you when you close your bedroom door. You may expand your answer to assure your child that you make love to be close to one another, but that you are using birth control because you don't want to have another baby at this time.

Such detailed information may seem premature to share with five- and six-year-old children, but it has been found that children absorb only that information that interests them. If your child becomes fidgety and distracted, wrap up the discussion and reopen it at another time. *One discussion is never enough.* It only introduces the child to the idea that *you are "askable."* The same information may be addressed in a number of ways in a number of circumstances according to the age, understanding, and maturity of the child.

Birth and the beginning of new life occur every fraction of a second. Refer to the Golden Opportunities interspersed throughout the book for examples of birth, such as raising plants from seedlings or hatching brine shrimp from dried eggs. The phenomenal event may be witnessed as a chick breaks through the shell of its egg or as the kitten pushes its way through the birth canal. Some parents are comfortable in observing nature's birthing process with their child. Others use video cassettes or library-loaned films designed specifically for children. Or, a parent may make reference to a neighbor who is pregnant. "I'll bet you noticed how big Mrs. Smith's tummy is getting. I bet you wondered why. When I was your age (four to six years), a lady in our neighborhood began to look just like Mrs. Smith. No one in my house ever spoke about it, and when I asked my mom she just said, "Because she's going to have a baby." I remember wondering how the baby got into her tummy and how it would get out. Now that I'm a mommy, I want you to know about many things that I wished I knew when I was your age. I want to help you to become smarter than I was so that you won't have to wonder about things that are special and beautiful."

You can ask Mrs. Smith if you and your child could pay her a visit. If there are no pregnant women in your life, you might ask your obstetrician if she or he has a patient who might let your child carefully touch her abdomen and listen to the baby's heart sounds by ear or with a stethoscope. You also can inquire at the local pet store or zoo if you may observe the birthing of an animal.

Mentally rehearsing strategies for initiating discussion about sexuality will increase your confidence to expand upon Golden Opportunities. Remember, they are everywhere! Leaf back through this book to trigger your imagination about the sexuality lessons related to a flower unfurling . . . sanitary items on a supermarket shelf . . . undergarments in a laundry basket . . . even a bowl of fruit and the baking of brownies. *You need not wait for your child to inquire.* Taking the initiative establishes your askability and eliminates the issue of the noninquiring child.

THE NONINQUIRING CHILD

Every seminar in sexuality reveals a parent who is concerned that their child has *not* asked a question about sex. "When should I tell her about the facts of life?" "If he doesn't ask, can I assume he isn't interested?" "Will I traumatize my child with information that she is not ready to accept?" After reading this book, you know the answers to these questions. From the moment of your child's birth, you should actively initiate information about sexuality. It's never too early to start. Accurate information is never harmful! Children will absorb as much information as they can comprehend and will ask again when they are ready to learn more.

Since sexual curiosity is a major theme of childhood, it is my belief that a so-called "noninquiring" child *has* asked about sexuality, but that his or her inquiry was not clearly framed because of shyness or poor verbal skills. There is also the possibility that the parent was distracted or misinterpreted the meaning behind an innocuous action or statement. For example, the three- or four-year-old boy who develops a bladder problem every time he leaves the house may be using the restroom as a resource for checking out the male anatomy. He has never inquired about his penis, but the time is right for a parent to initiate a discussion.

The four- or five-year-old who continues to touch his aunt's pregnant tummy has many unasked questions about a baby that lives inside a person's body. How does it eat? Does it sleep? Can it cry? How does it go to the bathroom?

A five- or six-year-old stares into a hatcher in wonderment as a chick pecks its way out of a shell. The child wonders aloud, "Wow, how did it get in there?" Without asking the child to clarify the comment, the parent delivers a long explanation about how the chick got into the shell. The child impatiently wanders away. If the parent had repeated the question exactly as stated by the child and followed it with the query, "How do you think it got there?" the child would have revealed that his curiosity was about how the chick got into the *hatcher* instead of residing with its mother in a nest like the bird outside of his bedroom window. The child was really wondering if he could take the egg outside his window from its nest and hatch it in his room.

"Listening with a third ear" requires hearing what may not have been stated. Sometimes a question is disguised or veiled as a statement. "Sheila's boyfriend really likes me a lot" may be a six-year-old's way of asking if it's OK for Sheila's boyfriend to kiss her on the mouth. A parent may ask, "How do you know that Sheila's boyfriend likes you a lot?" Such an inquiry invites the child to explain how the baby-sitter's boyfriend was expressing his affection toward the child.

The next question a parent asks is: What are the appropriate ages to introduce certain kinds of sexual information? The answer is that at different ages children will reveal different curiosities relevant to their stage of development. Since children's mental and physical maturity may widely vary, a working knowledge of these approximate stages is of great help.

THE AGES AND STAGES OF A CHILD'S SEXUAL QUESTIONING

What follows are questions most asked by children as they pass through the stages of sexual growth. You will see that a child's sexual curiosity about the same issue is repeated from one stage to the next. The maturing child may ask the same question as he or she did in early childhood, but now is seeking a more detailed answer. I suggest that you first answer the sample questions that follow to the best of your ability and in concert with your own values. Then consult the suggested answers that I have provided. In some instances, you may refer to a previous chapter for more detailed information about a particular subject.

Birth to 18 Months

We know that during the period from birth to 18 months the baby is learning about trust and love. Children explore their bodies and locate all their body parts. They receive a barrage of messages that will later be translated into what it means to be male or female. Satisfying the sensual needs of sucking, touching, holding, hearing, smelling, tasting, cooing, smiling, and communicating are life's earliest curiosities about sexuality. The ability of a baby boy to have an erection and an orgasm and a baby girl to experience a lubricated vagina affirms the natural and healthy expression of a child's sexuality. While babies may not be able to verbalize their questions, parents are constantly satisfying their child's curiosity by the tone of voice with which they communicate, along with facial expressions and the ease or tension they show in holding, bathing, cuddling, and feeding the baby. The baby's satisfaction through sucking, touching, and being fondled, along with the expectations of having its basic comforts met, form the rudiments of a child's sexual scripting. As the baby's sucking reflex is redirected from the bottle or breast to the cup, he or she experiences the first major milestone in his or her sexual development.

Rather than the child inquiring during this stage of development, it is parents who ask questions of themselves:

- Did I hold baby to my body during feeding?
- Did I focus my attention on the baby with eye contact and soft words of endearment?
- Did I touch, hug, and kiss the baby as expressions of appropriate intimacy?
- Did I make bath time a playful experience, and did I foster the baby's sensual appreciation with the application of baby oil and body massage?
- Did I display positive facial expressions as I changed the baby's soiled diaper?
- Did I confirm the baby's beauty with loving affirmations?
- Did I refer to the baby's anatomical parts by their proper names?
- Did I say "Yes" to each of baby's successes?

Eighteen Months to Three Years

The early preschool period from 18 months to three years is highlighted by a child's increasing sense of independence and curiosity.

Once weaned from the bottle, the next sexual milestone is toilet training. Children relish saying "No" during this stage as a way of establishing their own identity and taking charge of their own body. They develop new skills like walking, talking, socializing, and bowel control. Separation anxiety may be evidenced in a child's fear of being separated from a parent, as well as from his or her own body products, such as urine and feces. It's a time for children to discover the pleasure of exploring their genitals, and many explore their body products, as well. They are aware of their gender. They will identify with the parent of the same sex and ask questions about their parents' bodies. They may express a curiosity about the physiological differences between boys and girls and question the different postures required for each gender to urinate.

This is the beginning of the "What?, Why?, and How?" stage.

- "Why does the baby's belly button look funny?"
- "What are those bumps on your chest?"
- "How come he can stand up to make urine?"

It also ushers in the first inquiries about

- Where babies come from
- How babies get born

These early questions require simple answers:

- "The baby's belly button will soon look like yours and mine (observe both). When the baby was inside Mommy's uterus, it got its food through a tube (umbilical cord), which connected the baby's belly button to my uterus. Now that the baby no longer lives inside my uterus, it eats food with its mouth like you and me. It doesn't need the tube anymore. The little end of the tube will soon disappear, and the baby's belly button will look just like ours."
- "The bumps on my chest are called breasts. When you get to be big like me and cousin Jill, you will grow breasts, too."
- "A boy stands up to make urine because it's easier for him to direct his urine from his penis into the toilet. A girl makes urine from a place inside her vulva, and it's easier for her to direct her urine into the toilet by sitting down." (Mother may show child where the opening for urine [the urethra] is located in the vulva.)

Three to Six Years

During these years, children affirm their gender identity. They passed through the Oedipal stage of being competitive with their parent of the same sex and now choose to emulate that parent's behavior. Their play is imaginative or magical; they act out their impressions of male and female roles and behavior. Often play is so fanciful that it may be misinterpreted as lies.

A three-year-old is interested in marriage and may propose to either parent, thinking that people can be married to either sex. By the age of six, they are still fascinated with marriage, but they would make such a proposal to someone of the opposite sex, often a relative. From five to seven years, they test heterosexual marriage by playing house.

They have a keen interest in where babies come from and how they get in and out of a mommy's tummy. Even though a parent may have explained the birth process many times, the child may still think that a baby can be bought in a store or that it grows from a seed and enters the world via Mommy's navel. They are often intrigued with their own belly buttons and ask many questions related to its size, shape, and function. Their interest in the anatomical differences between boys and girls increases. Their curiosity is evidenced by their desire to play doctor and "show-me" games.

By ages three and four, they may express or display a fear of their anatomical differences. "What happened to my penis?" (if circumcised or uncircumcised) and "Why don't I have a penis?" are typical queries. The noninquiring child may clasp his or her genitals. In times of stress, boys are prone to grasp their penis. Children often compare their anatomy by staring at or touching their parents' genitals.

They have intense curiosity about bathroom activities and often call one another names related to body products and genitals. They generally ignore sex differences in choosing friends for play, but boys may reject so-called girls' games, such as playing with dolls.

By the time they are six, they may play doctor and take one another's rectal temperature or place objects into their orifices, as well as expose themselves in play or in schoolrooms. It is an important time to emphasize appropriate and inappropriate touch and rules for modesty and propriety. The "What if" game described in Chapter 7 can be a great help here.

Again and again, questions are raised about pregnancy and birth, and children may express their desire for a new baby in the family. By the sixth year, they are less interested in bathroom activities and more aware of the natural differences between boys and girls. They begin to associate, often with some anxiety, the good feelings they have from touching their genitals or rubbing their body against objects or people. This is the time to reassure them that self-pleasuring is fine but that sex-play, especially with older persons, is not OK.

Parents' sexual values are challenged during these years when children ask such questions as:

- Jimmy says those are the baby's balls. What are they for?
- Why can't I go to the bathroom with Daddy?
- How come Rebecca's penis fell off?
- Why can't I have a baby?
- My vagina feels good and tingles when I rock on my horse.
- Billy said Jane is a cunt. What is that?
- Why can't Sammy take my temperature? You do.
- Does it hurt to have a baby?
- How do babies eat from their mommy's breasts?
- Can I drink milk from your breasts, too?
- Can I marry my brother and have a baby?

Jimmy says those are the baby's balls. What are they for?

Balls is one of those incorrect words that people sometimes use to refer to the small sac that hangs behind the penis, right next to a boy or man's body. (A more complete answer for a more mature child may be expanded.) Inside the sac are two small round bumps that may feel like balls. These are called testicles. They make sperm when a boy gets to be as big as Cousin Jerry (between ages 11 and 13). Sperm are what the man puts into a woman's vagina through the penis to meet a woman's egg and make a baby.

Why can't I go to the bathroom with Daddy?

Daddy prefers that you don't go with him to the bathroom now that you are getting to be big. Daddy and I feel more comfortable doing private things (like urinating and showering) in private places. *To expand the explanation:* If the door is closed, that means it is a private time. As you keep getting bigger, you will want more private time, too. The rule is: When the door is closed, knock first, and if the private time is finished, you may enter.

How come Rebecca's penis fell off?

Rebecca's penis did not fall off. Rebecca is a girl, and all girls and mommies are born with their own special part of their body called a vulva. A vulva does many of the good things that a penis does, but it looks altogether different. If Rebecca were a boy or a daddy, she would have been born with a penis. *To expand the explanation:* A boy uses his penis to urinate and to touch for good feelings. When he's grown up, the penis helps make a baby. Inside a girl's vulva is an opening (urethra) through which the urine passes. A special spot (clitoris) feels good to touch and another opening, called a vagina, is for making babies.

Why can't I have a baby?

You can't have a baby because you are not big enough. When you get to be as big as Cousin Rosa or me, you will have grown breasts on the outside of your body and you will have eggs (not like chicken eggs) inside your body that can make a baby when they come in contact with the sperm from a man's penis. It's best to wait to have a baby until you are grown up like Mommy and Daddy.

My vagina feels good and tingles when I rock on my horse.

Your vagina feels good and tingles when you ride on the rocking horse because the special place inside your vulva (the clitoris) is supposed to feel good when it is touched. It is being rubbed as you rock back and forth. I'm glad that it feels good and tingly, but if you rock long and hard, it may become red and irritated. The sunshine feels good and tingly, too, but too much sun can give you a hurting sunburn.

Billy said Jane is a cunt. What is that?

When Billy called Jane a cunt he was being very rude. He probably didn't even know what he was saying. *Cunt* is a wrong word for vagina, the special place between a woman's legs (inside her vulva) through which a baby passes to be born. *You may expand the answer:* When a man and woman make love, the man or woman places the man's penis into the vagina and they both get good and tingly feelings.

Why can't Sammy take my temperature? You do.

It is not a good idea for Sammy to put anything inside your anus. Sammy is only playing, and he is not as gentle as me or Dr. Smith. When he takes your temperature, he may hurt the inside of your body, and the thermometer can break and hurt you, too. *You may expand:* It can be hurtful to put any object, except the gentle touch of your finger, into any opening in your body.

Does it hurt to have a baby?

Having a baby can hurt as the baby inside the mommy's uterus pushes down with his or her head so that it can stretch the mommy's vagina and pass through it to be born. Mommies learn how to help the baby push through the vagina. Some doctors give a mommy medicine so that she doesn't even feel the baby being born. Usually there is so much joy when the baby is born that the mommy quickly forgets about the discomfort.

How do babies eat from their mommy's breast?

Only when a mommy has a baby do her breasts become filled with milk. When the baby sucks this milk from tiny holes in the mother's nipple, the mother's breasts make more milk. The more the baby drinks, the more the breasts fill with milk. *You may add:* If a mother chooses not to breast-feed her baby, the milk dries up and the mommy's breasts return to their normal size.

Can I drink milk from your breasts, too?

When you were a little baby you did drink milk from my breasts, just like your sister. Now that you are a big boy with big boy teeth, it may hurt Mommy's breasts. Big boys and big girls don't drink from baby bottles either; they drink from a cup or glass, like a mommy or daddy. (You may want to demonstrate how you express milk from your breasts in making a reserve bottle, and you may satisfy your child's curiosity by providing a sample of the milk in a cup.)

Can I marry my brother and have a baby?

Brothers and sisters are not allowed to get married or to make love or to have babies together. It is against the law. *You may continue:* It is against the law for parents or relatives to marry and neither they nor their grown-up friends can make love to children. If any one of these people ever touches you in a private place, please tell Mommy and Daddy and remind the person that it is wrong and against the law.

Seven to Nine Years

By the age of seven, a child's curiosity about the physical difference between the sexes is usually resolved. Since children at this time are less verbally inquisitive, it has been considered a time of sexual latency by followers of the Freudian school of psychology. Modern sexologists believe, however, that *this stage is a time for sexual introspection, and that it is vitally linked to a child's growing awareness of his or her sexual organs and their functions.* Curiosity about the opposite sex is evidenced by their deliberate segregation in play and teasing boys and girls who become friends. By the age of nine, play with the opposite sex may lead to kissing and petting. Horseplay between the sexes provides opportunities for children's increased need to be touched. It's a period when children tell dirty jokes, use foul words, giggle provocatively, create crude poems, and invent secret languages and code words. They are less apt to tolerate "tall tales" and now seek logical answers to previously accepted "truths." While many children hesitate to uncover the realities about Santa Claus and the Tooth Fairy, this is the stage of life where it becomes imperative to dispel myths, especially those related to anatomy, intercourse, and the birth process. Marriage as a union between one man and one woman with the goal to have a child and live in a home becomes fully comprehensible.

Learning about their changing bodies through self-exploration, masturbation, the media, magazines, and the exchange of sex information and sex-play with same-sex friends increases by the age of nine. This is a period of expressed modesty and the need for increased privacy. Children are particularly self-conscious as they approach puberty, and they desperately need affection and affirmation from their adult world.

Typical questions asked at this time are:

- Is my penis big enough?
- What is a blow job?
- Will I ever grow tall?
- How can you tell if a girl has her period?
- Does everyone masturbate?
- Do you and Dad have intercourse?
- When a girl gets her period, does she bleed every day?
- Does she wear a sanitary pad every day?
- If you get a divorce, can you still have a baby?
- What is a homosexual?
- Do homosexuals have babies?
- What is butt-fucking?
- Do I have a seed in me?

Is my penis big enough?

Your penis is just the right size for your body. As you grow older, your hands will grow larger, as well as your feet, your nose, and your penis. Boys often tease one another about the size of their penis. When a penis is soft, it may look small, but when it gets hard (through masturbation, need to urinate, stress, change in temperature) it can expand to nearly twice its size before it gets soft again. It's like blowing up an *unbreakable* balloon and then letting out the air.

What is a blow job?

A *blow job* is a slang word for oral sex, a way in which some people choose to make love. Oral sex occurs when a woman places a man's penis in her mouth and licks it or sucks it. A man can provide oral sex by choosing to kiss, lick, or suck a woman's vulva and clitoris. Because the germs from AIDS may enter a person's mouth during oral sex, adults often cover the penis with a rubber sheath (condom) that looks like a deflated balloon. (The child may find the notion of oral sex repugnant and question why people do this. You may explain that some grown-up people enjoy this form of lovemaking, while other grown-up people choose not to engage in oral sex.)

Will I ever grow tall?

Everybody has a different body clock. Some people have a clock that goes faster than others. There are growth hormones in your body that will soon begin to stimulate your body clock to move faster. Once you start to grow hair above your penis and your voice begins to change, your body will produce hormones that will help your body grow taller. You probably will grow to be about the same size as mom and me.

How can you tell if a girl has her period?

You really can't tell if a girl has her period unless she chooses to tell you. She will look exactly as she does every day, except she will wear a sanitary pad or a tampon (which she changes in the bathroom every three to four hours) so that there is no odor from the collection of the menstrual flow.

Does everyone masturbate?

No, everyone doesn't purposely pleasure themselves, but almost everyone, at one time or another, has felt the pleasure of rubbing their genitals against the bed linen or pressing their thighs tightly together or directing the water spray on the penis and testicles or vulva and clitoris. People who choose to masturbate usually use their hands for self-pleasuring.

Do you and Dad have intercourse?

Sure we do. Usually when we close the door to our room for privacy, Daddy and I make love to each other because it is fun and it brings us pleasure. We also can have intercourse in order to make a baby. Right now we choose not to have children, so we use birth control to keep Daddy's sperm from meeting my egg.

When a girl gets her period, does she bleed every day? Does she always have to wear a sanitary pad?

No. Girls only bleed about three to six days out of every month. In the beginning, a girl may even skip a month or two between one period and the next. It takes about a year before her periods are regular. Girls only have to wear sanitary napkins or tampons on those few days each month that they are menstruating, to catch the menstrual flow.

If you get a divorce, can you still have a baby?

Yes. Even people who are not married can get a baby if they have intercourse without using birth control. It's much easier for a mother to be married when she has a baby so that she has another person to help with the baby's care.

What is a homosexual?

A homosexual is a person who chooses to have sex only with another person of the same sex. A heterosexual is someone who prefers to have sexual relations with someone of the opposite sex.

Do homosexuals have babies?

If a lesbian woman were to have intercourse with a homosexual or heterosexual man, without using birth control, she could become pregnant when his sperm meets her egg inside her tube. But gay men and lesbian women choose to have sex only with a person of the same gender, so there is no way for the sperm to fertilize the egg and for the woman to become pregnant. Gay men and lesbian women can adopt a baby and raise it as their own child. (A more complete explanation may include the possibility of artificial insemination.)

What is butt-fucking?

Butt-fucking is the slang term for anal sex. When people choose to have anal sex, one partner places his penis into the anus of the other person. It is considered an unsafe form of lovemaking because the anus is a tender area and can become irritated when it is stretched. It is also an area of the body that contains many germs because it is the opening through which you move your bowels. People who choose to have anal sex should always wear a rubber sheath (condom) to cover their penis and protect it from spreading germs or the virus of AIDS.

Do I have a seed in me?

No, not yet. A boy's body doesn't begin to make seeds or sperm cells until he's about 11 or 12 or even 15 years old. He usually knows when he has begun to make sperm cells when a white liquid called semen comes out of his erect penis. This usually first happens during his sleep and is called a wet dream.

Nine to Twelve—Prepuberty

This stage of development may be particularly awkward. The growth hormones naturally begin to awaken two years earlier for girls than for boys. It may be a time of shyness and modesty. Both sexes are keenly interested in their body changes, especially the development of their secondary sex characteristics, such as their breasts budding, the penis growing wider and longer, the growth of pubic hair, acne, and voice change. The onset of the menstrual cycle and nocturnal emissions are heralded as rites of passage. Some preteens are painfully self-conscious about their body changes and often use teasing as a form of defense. They are sensitive to the media idols who define "handsome" and "pretty," and begin to have crushes on members of the opposite sex. Experimental same-sex play may be actively engaged in as a means of exploring their sexuality (see Chapter 7). While boys may discuss their masturbating experience with friends and even engage in mutual masturbation, girls are generally too inhibited or embarrassed to discuss their experiences with anyone. Sexual fantasies may be a source of stress for both sexes. "Am I normal?" is the nagging question that causes prepubescent anxiety.

Because of the wide variance of children's physical and emotional development at this age, as well as myriad of environmental influences, concerns and questions about sexuality may vary widely from child to child. Questions may range from the ridiculous to the sublime:

- Why haven't I gotten my period yet?
- Is it weird to dream about naked people?
- Does intercourse hurt?
- What is an orgasm?
- Can you get pregnant without having intercourse?
- When a man puts his penis in a woman's vagina, can he urinate inside her?
- What's a virgin?
- Where is the cherry?
- What is birth control?
- Can a boy have intercourse if he hasn't any sperm?
- What is menopause?
- Do boys have menstrual periods?
- What's VD?
- What are fraternal twins?
- What is rape?

Why haven't I gotten my period yet?

Because we each develop according to the timing of our personal body clock, each girl gets her period at a different time. Some girls begin to menstruate as early as 8 years of age, and others as late as 15 years of age. It depends on your hormones, your body fat and weight, and even the climate in which you live. You can expect your period about six months to a year after your breasts begin to develop and you begin to grow hair around your vulva.

Is it weird to dream about naked people?

No. Dreaming is normal and healthy. When we sleep, our mind is free to think about anything. Our dreams are a safe way of venturing into activities that we would never engage in when we are awake. Often our fantasies are about relatives or friends, only because they are familiar pictures that our mind is able to develop while we sleep. It's difficult for the mind to develop dreams about strangers.

Does intercourse hurt?

Sometimes the first time a woman has intercourse it may be uncomfortable, as the walls of the woman's vagina are stretched to accommodate the penis. If both partners are loving and gentle and have discussed their desire to make love with one another, the experience is usually pleasurable for the man and woman. When both partners take their time in pleasuring one another before having intercourse, the woman's vagina will become moist. This moisture is nature's way of helping the penis to enter the vagina.

What is an orgasm?

A person can experience an orgasm (which only lasts for a few seconds) from masturbating, sexual intercourse, and even from reading or viewing erotic materials. An orgasm occurs at the height of sexual excitement (climax) for both a man and a woman. Orgasm happens when the muscles and the nerves in the penis and testicles of men and in the clitoris, vagina, and uterus of women contract and relax many times until the body completely relaxes in a state of pleasure. The man's penis will release (ejaculate) a teaspoon or two of a white fluid called semen, and the walls of the vagina will become moist (lubricate). Some people say an orgasm is a wonderful warm and tingly sensation that surges through your body from your head to your toes.

Can you get pregnant without having intercourse?

Yes. If a girl has gotten her first menstrual period and her eggs have matured to travel from her ovaries through her fallopian tubes (ovulation), she is capable of becoming pregnant if a man deposits his semen (ejaculate) *near* the opening of her vagina. Sperm can swim from outside the vagina into the uterus to fertilize an egg. A woman also can get pregnant when a doctor injects a man's semen through a syringe and into a woman's vagina when she is ovulating. This is called artificial insemination.

When a man puts his penis in a woman's vagina, can he urinate inside her?

No. When a man's penis gets hard enough to enter a woman's vagina, it can release only sperm (semen). It cannot release urine at the same time.

What is a virgin?

A virgin is a man or a woman who has never had sexual intercourse.

Where is the cherry?

Cherry is a slang word for the hymen, which is a flexible, thin or thick tissue that covers the opening of the vagina. The hymen may have a small opening through which the menstrual discharge flows or it may have many openings from natural causes like athletics. The expression "breaking the cherry" may refer to a person's first experience with intercourse, especially if the stretching of the hymen leads to some spotting of blood.

What is birth control?

Birth control is a method people use when they wish to have sexual intercourse without getting pregnant. Every method is designed to keep the sperm from meeting the egg. There are many forms of birth control, like the birth control pill, diaphragm, sponge, condom, and jellies, creams, and suppositories placed in the vagina to kill sperm. (A chart describing all birth control methods can be found in the Appendix.)

Can a boy have intercourse if he hasn't any sperm?

Yes. A boy can place his erect penis into a girl's vagina even before he is able to make sperm. Since intercourse is a special way for two adults to express their love for one another, it is not a good idea for children to make play out of a beautiful grown-up experience.

What is menopause?

Menopause happens to a woman at 45 or 55 when her menstruation cycle slowly stops. When a woman no longer menstruates, she is unable to become pregnant, but she can, of course, still enjoy intercourse.

Do boys have menstrual periods?

No. Only girls and women menstruate. Menstruation "tells" them that they are capable of having babies. Boys and men know that they are capable of making babies with a woman when they have a wet dream. A wet dream happens at night when they are sleeping (nocturnal emission). A boy's penis becomes hard and he ejaculates sperm in the semen that has been stored in his testicles. Often a boy or man will experience a dream while he ejaculates.

What is VD?

VD is the abbreviation for venereal disease. We now refer to venereal diseases as Sexually Transmitted Diseases (STDs) because these are diseases that people catch from one another when they exchange body fluids during sexual intercourse or by kissing and sucking sexual parts, such as the penis, the vulva, clitoris, and the anus. Some STDs are herpes, AIDS, gonorrhea, and syphilis. People who use condoms along with spermicidal creams and jellies are less likely to get STDs when they make love.

What are fraternal twins?

Fraternal twins are produced when two separate eggs from the mother's ovaries are fertilized by two separate sperm from the man's semen. The mother's uterus provides a separate sac (placenta) for each of the babies to grow in during the nine months of pregnancy. Each baby is attached to its placenta by its separate cord (umbilical) and separate navels. Each baby's blood, food, oxygen, water, and waste products flow through the cord to the placenta. When the babies are born, they do not look alike (identical) and may even be different sexes. They may not have the same blood type or skin coloring. They are two babies born at the same time to the same mother and father.

What is rape?

Rape occurs when someone physically forces another person to have sexual intercourse when it is against that person's will. Rape is against the law. People who rape are mentally ill. The person who is raped is always a victim and never to blame. The person who commits the rape is always guilty.

Twelve to Sixteen Years—Early Adolescence

These are years of tumultuous hormonal changes. There is a wide variance between the sexual maturity of boys and girls, as well as among children of the same sex. The range between 12 and 14 can be so dramatic that it is often hard to predict the concerns that may arise. What makes it more problematic is that the earlier developer may not be any more emotionally mature than the later developer.

Boys reach their growth spurt at about 15 and girls at about age 12, so each sex is likely to feel physically awkward in the other's company. Questions about petting, masturbation, homosexuality, intercourse, and social skills are likely to be broached. During this time, teens are torn between their desire to achieve and their need for peer acceptance, as well as between their drive for independence and their continued need for parental approval and guidance. Girls often have questions about peer acceptance, while boys usually question their assertiveness skills, masculine identity, and erotic feelings.

As teens search for their individuality, they keep falling back to the conformity of the group for fear of being unacceptable or unpopular. They begin to reject standards set by adults and abide by values and double standards dictated by their small same-sex peer group. Their preoccupation with same-sex cliques is the forerunner to seeking close heterosexual ties.

Falling in love, especially for girls, may be confined to a crush on an older person as they rehearse and fantasize about a love-sex relationship. Early adolescents often live a fabled existence in which they feel immune to all risks such as unplanned pregnancy and even death. Their ability to make choices beyond today and tomorrow is limited, and they haven't yet developed the skills to make long-term decisions. Therefore, the need to address choices, responsibility, and alternatives to impulsive self-fulfillment is as important as providing the basic facts of life.

Typical questions that early adolescents usually ask are:

- Why am I getting breasts like a girl?
- How come I haven't had a wet dream?
- When will my voice stop squeaking?

- Will I still be a virgin if I use tampons?
- Are boys sexier than girls?
- Is it weird to be in love with Mr. Weiss?
- Do you think it's romantic that Romeo would kill himself for Juliet?
- Am I going to be a lesbian if Jackie and I touched each other's breasts and vagina?
- Is there any way I can make my penis/breasts larger?
- When a boy gets a hard-on, does he have to "cum" or else he'll get "blue balls"?
- Can your penis get hard for no special reason?
- If only one sperm out of millions fertilizes the egg, what happens to the rest of the sperm?
- What's the clitoris?

Why am I getting breasts like a girl?

All girls and boys develop breasts as they mature. Boys' breasts usually are firmed by muscles, but more than 25 percent of boys develop enlarged breasts and nipple sensitivity during their early adolescence. While this may make you feel self-conscious and anxious, this tissue will soon turn to muscle and the swelling will disappear. Exercises with barbells and push-ups will speed up the process.

How come I haven't had a wet dream?

Not every boy experiences his first ejaculation of sperm with a nighttime orgasm or a nocturnal emission. Many boys, about a year after they start to develop pubic hair (10 to 15 years of age) will have a wet dream during sleep while dreaming about sex. Others, who relieve their body of sperm by masturbating to orgasm during the day or night, may never or rarely have wet dreams.

When will my voice stop squeaking?

As your body begins to produce sex hormones, your voice box grows and affects the pitch of your speech. It's kind of embarrassing when your voice fluctuates from squeaking high to bass in a matter of moments. It takes about two years for boys to adjust to their vocal chord changes. Girls' voices change also, but it's not as noticeable.

Will I still be a virgin if I use tampons?
Sure you will. A virgin is someone who has not had a penis enter her vagina. A tampon is a hygiene product that, when inserted into your vagina to absorb the menstrual flow, will not steal away your virginity.

Are boys sexier than girls?
No. Boys and girls are equally able to enjoy their sexual feelings, from masturbation to petting, but for generations girls have been socialized to believe that only boys get good sexual feelings and that it's a girl's job to control a boy's sexual drive. As the double standard begins to fade, girls are discovering their potential for sexual enjoyment.

Is it weird to be in love with Mr. Weiss?
No. It's normal to feel as though you love a man who is as kind and caring as Mr. Weiss is. In fact, I can remember having a crush on my math teacher when I was your age. It shouldn't make you nervous, because you won't act out your fantasies about this love affair. It is your way of deciding what traits you most admire in people. Later, when you feel more comfortable with the opposite sex, you may look for these same traits in a boyfriend.

Do you think it's romantic that Romeo would kill himself for Juliet?
Not only do I *not* think it is romantic, I think it is stupid. No one's happiness and desire to live should rest upon another person's love and affection. Some operas and stories romanticize suicide for the sake of love, but nothing is more sacred than life. The world is filled with people to love. Even when a person feels that his or her heart will never be repaired from a broken love affair, there is always another person whose love is waiting to be discovered. Suicide never mends a broken heart; it only causes deeper pain for everyone involved. Suicide is forever. A person never wakes up from suicide. His or her life is ended.

Am I going to be a lesbian if Jackie and I touched each other's breasts and vagina?

No. It's not unusual for teens of the same sex to sexually arouse one another. It is a way of learning how your body responds to the touch of another person. As you feel more comfortable with yourself and people of the opposite sex, you will transfer these good feelings to a special boyfriend.

Is there any way I can make my penis/breasts larger?

No. Every person comes packaged in a way that is perfectly designed to meet the individual. There are no exercises, pills, or creams that can make your breasts (or penis) larger. The size of all your body parts is determined by heredity. They will probably grow to be about the same size as Daddy's and mine, and we have been perfectly happy with all our body parts.

When a boy gets a hard-on, does he have to "cum" or else he'll get "blue balls?"

No. Once the penis becomes erect, it can become relaxed again without having to ejaculate. A boy will not get "blue balls." He merely has to think of things other than sex or involve himself in another activity for the erection to disappear. If the need to ejaculate continues, he can relieve the sexual tension by masturbating to orgasm. By the way, a woman is capable of the same heightened sexual sensation with tension felt in her pelvic region. The remedy to relieve the tension is the same for women as men.

Can your penis get hard for no special reason?

Yes. The penis sometimes appears to have a mind of its own. It is normal for the penis occasionally to become erect when a boy least expects it. Every boy has had an embarrassing experience when his penis became erect while sitting in a math class or dancing or watching TV.

If only one sperm out of millions fertilizes one egg, what happens to the rest of the sperm?

Millions of sperm are killed as they struggle to reach the egg.

Hundreds of thousands swim into the woman's uterus and remain alive for two or even three days until they finally die and pass out of the woman's body.

What is the clitoris?

It is a small, sensitive, rounded "buttonlike" female sex organ that is located toward the top and inside the inner lips of the vagina. The clitoris is the sexual pleasure center for girls and women when it is touched or rubbed.

Late Adolescence—Sixteen Years and Older

This phase marks a major thrust towards independence and mature sexual identity. Sexuality is clearly the central theme of these years, as teens question their feelings, attitudes, skills, goals, and ability to be lovable and successful. The double standard and peer pressure often place teens in a double bind in deciding whether to accept or reject sexual advances. By late adolescence, teens are able to think in conceptual, future-oriented terms. They become less ego-focused and develop a higher capacity for social/moral judgment. It is during this time that teens tackle the weightiest questions about human sexuality and the ethical aspects of relationships. Premarital sex, contraception, planned and unplanned pregnancy, sexually transmitted diseases, and cohabitation outside of marriage challenge their frame of reference.

Words like *love, sex, guilt, respect, equality, morality, trust, sin, commitment, honesty,* and *intimacy* are defined and redefined as teens establish their sexual values. They look to respected adults in their life for honest dialogue about sex-role expectations and responsible sexual behavior:

- How can I say "No"?
- Is everybody doing "IT"?
- How do you know when you are in love?
- How can you be popular without "going all the way"?
- Can you get AIDS from oral sex?
- What is sodomy?
- What's the best form of birth control?

- How can you tell if you have VD?
- What is an abortion and how can you get one?
- How do you know if you're a good lover?
- Can you have sex without being in love?
- Am I weird if I'm not interested in sex?
- Why can't I sleep with my boyfriend in your home? We sleep together at college.
- What and where is the G-spot?
- What exactly is "safer sex"?

How can I say "No"?

"I really like being with you. I enjoy being kissed and held and cuddled, but please don't pressure me to have intercourse. I'm not ready, and I don't want to spoil our wonderful relationship. If and when I am ready, I'll let you know."

Is everybody doing "IT"?

No. In fact, more people are not doing "IT" now because of their fear of sexually transmitted diseases such as herpes and AIDS. People are becoming more creative in pleasuring one another with erotic *outercourse* and are saving *intercourse* for a time when they feel more ready.

How do you know when you're in love?

Love makes you feel happy, secure, and more sure of yourself. You feel a strong desire to be close to one another and express your emotions through close physical contact. You take pleasure in looking at one another and are proud to be together in the company of others. You care about one another's feelings and well-being. You support each other's values as well as one another's desire to achieve success and recognition. You trust one another to share secrets without the fear of criticism or ridicule. You may feel as though you have fallen in love many times before you finally choose your love-mate for marriage.

How can you be popular without "going all the way"?

All the surveys show that popular people do not "go all the

way." People who are popular have a ready smile, a friendly person-ality, a good sense of humor, and are usually successful at school or work. They are busy people who enjoy activities and are involved in projects to help others or to improve their environment. Popular people have a knack for remembering to say nice things to people who deserve compliments and earn the friendship and respect of others without having to sacrifice their sexual values.

Can you get AIDS from oral sex?

Yes. You can get AIDS when any body fluid containing the virus of AIDS is transferred from one person into the body of another. Women providing oral sex to men should use a condom to protect themselves from swallowing semen or the clear pre-ejaculate fluid. Men providing oral sex to women should use the spermicidal nonoxynol-9 on the lips of the vagina, along with a small, thin square of rubber (dentist's dam) or a female condom stretched over the vagina to guard against swallowing vaginal secretions. *You may expand your answer:* Even French kissing (deep kissing or tongue kissing), where there is the exchange of saliva from one person to another, is considered risky, especially if one partner has bleeding gums or an injury in his or her mouth. Dry kissing, without the exchange of saliva, on any part of the body, except the anus, or of the penis, is considered safe from the transfer of any body fluids from one person into the body of another. [Addendum: While *at this time* there is no proof that anyone has contracted AIDS through the saliva of kissing, we do know that the virus of AIDS, in low concentration, has been found in saliva.]

What is sodomy?

Sodomy is a legal term that usually means that a person has intercourse by placing his penis into the anus of another person (anal intercourse). In some states, sodomy is also defined as a person placing his penis into the mouth of another (oral sex) as a form of intercourse.

What's the best form of birth control?

The best form of birth control is the method with which you

feel most comfortable and which you will use correctly. The birth control pill is the form of birth control that provides the highest form of pregnancy prevention, by suspending the process of ovulation. The diaphragm and the sponge are barriers that a woman inserts into her vagina each time she has intercourse. The condom, used with spermicidal jelly and cream, offers the best protection against sexually transmitted diseases and is recommended as an additional form of protection regardless of what other measure of birth control a person uses. Of course, the safest and surest form of birth control is abstaining, which means not having intercourse at all. (Refer to chart of birth control methods in Appendix).

How can you tell if you have VD?

Venereal disease or sexually transmitted diseases (STDs) can be detected sometimes by a visual examination or laboratory test. To test for syphilis, herpes, and the antibodies of AIDS, blood is collected from a vein and tested. To test for gonorrhea and herpes, a culture is made from the lesion to detect the exact organism. Some STDs can be detected by placing a sample of the disease's secretion on a slide and examining it under a microscope. Almost all forms of STDs can be cured with medication. The lesions of herpes may be lessened, but not cured, with a medication. AIDS is *incurable,* and even the negative results of a blood test cannot guarantee that a person's body is permanently free of the virus. The virus may incubate in the body for months or years before detected by a blood test.

What is an abortion and how can you get one?

Abortion is the stopping of a pregnancy. A woman's body may naturally stop the pregnancy if she has a miscarriage or a spontaneous abortion, or she may choose to end the pregnancy by mechanical means. In this case, a doctor will assist in removing the pregnancy from the uterus by using a suction method of aspiration or by means of medications and instruments. At this time, anyone can legally receive a medically provided abortion. *You may choose to add:* While early abortions are safe and legal, it is easier and wiser to use contraceptives to prevent an unplanned pregnancy. Abortion is *not* a form of birth control.

How do you know if you are a good lover?

Good lovers take equal joy in giving and receiving pleasure. By gently guiding one another's hands and telling each other the caresses and kisses that are pleasurable, each person has a sense of their "love-ability." Ask your partner about his or her pleasure zones. Each person has his or her personal and unique style for lovemaking.

Can you have sex without being in love?

The factual answer is "Yes." Many people choose to have sex for the pleasure of the activity, to release sexual tension, and for a wide variety of reasons other than love. *Whenever possible it is wise to include an addendum about safe sex:* People who care about their own health and that of others use birth control and safe-sex techniques to avoid pregnancy and STDs.

Am I weird if I'm not interested in sex?

No. Celibacy (choosing not to have sex) is every person's right and may be a phase of life or a life-style a person chooses to follow. Sexual energy may be released through masturbation, physical activity, creative endeavor, mental stimulation, or spiritual devotion. Sexual activity should never be entered into unless it is by mutual consent.

Why can't I sleep with my boyfriend in your home? We sleep together at college.

My home is my sanctuary, and therefore I have the right to make the rules for those living or visiting with me. I have no objection to your testing your love relationship on campus, but I am uncomfortable with the arrangement in my home. I respect your right to live as you choose as an independent adult. I ask that you grant me the same right.

What and where is the G-spot?

The G-spot is named for Grafenberg, a German doctor who in

1944 discovered in some women a sexually sensitive area (erogenous zone) located deep within the upper or front wall of the vagina. It wasn't researched, and women didn't discuss it until the 1980s. Some women believe that when they are stimulated in this area, they can experience an orgasm and actually ejaculate a clear, odorless fluid similar but different in color and consistency from a man's ejaculate. Since the theory has only recently been described by some women, it is not yet accepted as fact by everybody who studies sexuality. *You may add:* The thought is that even if the theory is correct, the G-spot may not be sensitive in all women. The danger is that some women may search for but not feel the G-spot and then believe that they are not normal.

What exactly is "safer sex"?

Safer sex involves engaging in loving intimacy while avoiding intercourse. It may include activities such as fantasy, fondling, erotic videos, phone sex, caressing, kissing, and sucking the breasts and nipples, rubbing the penis between the breasts, thighs, or armpits, whispering erotic dialogue to one another, or engaging in exhibitionism and creative playfulness with one another. When oral sex and intercourse are included, it means eroticizing condoms so that they become an exciting and integral part of the sex act.

In completing this section, dozens of additional questions come to mind from the hundreds of anonymous queries submitted by parents and children at sexuality seminars I have conducted in past years. This sampling is a motivational introduction to the wonderful world of inquiry waiting to be discovered. My guess is that once you see how gratifying it is to satisfy your child's curiosity with accurate information that reflects your value system, you will continue to discover Golden Opportunities for continued communication. And once your children recognize your askability, they'll find the courage to ask soulful questions such as:

- How can I be in charge of my feelings?
- How do you know which people you can really trust?
- How can I be more popular?

- How can I develop the courage to say "No" and the confidence to say "Yes"?
- How can I be like everyone else and still act as though I'm the first, the last, the best, the original?

THE JOURNEY ENDS AS THE MISSION BEGINS

Congratulations! You have just completed a personal sexual journey. You are now capable of creating a new legacy for your child. You will find that raising your child to be sexually healthy is an evolutionary process in which the entire family learns, grows, and benefits. As a parent, you become a knowledgeable and trusted resource for your child. As a spouse, you expand intimate communication and increase your repertoire of sexual information and pleasure. Together, the sexually evolved family bonds in a common mission to eliminate sin, guilt, inequity, fear, and embarrassment from life's most rewarding pleasurable potential.

A child born into an environment of warmth, honesty, trust, acceptance, and knowledge will mature into an adult who can love himself or herself and others, joyfully embracing all of life's blessings. What better endowment can you give your children than the ability to respect, and value themselves? Who is better suited to bestow this gift of love than you? And when is there a better time to begin this mission than now?

PERSONAL MESSAGE FROM THE AUTHOR

In sharing this book, our lives have touched in a spiritual sense. I welcome an opportunity to know you more personally and invite you to write to me expressing your views, comments, or questions. We become one another's teachers as we extend our hands in friendship. You may write to me at:

The Sex, Health, Education Center
12550 Biscayne Boulevard
North Miami, Florida 33181

*

Appendix

Pictorial Answers to Fundamental Questions
About Sex and Reproduction

FEMALE REPRODUCTIVE SYSTEM

Pituitary Gland: The small gland that receives its messages from the hypothalamus (at the base of the brain) to release hormones through the bloodstream that signal the ovaries to produce estrogen and progesterone. This gland and its hormones control the menstrual cycle and cause a tiny egg to ripen in an ovary.

Ovaries: There are two located at the end of the fallopian tubes at each side of the uterus. Each contains thousands of tiny egg sacs that are present at birth but do not mature until the first menses. From that time on, once a month, an egg ripens, breaks out of its sac, and travels from the ovary into the fallopian tube. It may take months or even years before the cycle occurs like clockwork every month. This monthly event, called ovulation, continues until a woman reaches menopause and the ovaries no longer produce eggs.

Fallopian Tubes: Two funnel-like tubes with fringe-like "fingers" (fimbria) that curl around and almost reach each ovary. The fimbria draw a ripened egg from an ovary into the fallopian tube. Fertilization usually takes place during the egg's four- to six-day journey to the uterus.

Uterus: A hollow, pear-shaped organ that connects on top to the fallopian tubes and dips at the lower end, at its mouth or cervix, into the vagina. Each month the uterine lining thickens with a rich blood supply to nourish a fertilized egg as it develops into a baby. When an unfertilized egg enters the uterus, the lining is not needed. The egg disintegrates and passes out of the body, along with the lining. This happens about every 28 days with a menstrual flow that passes from the uterus, through the cervix, and out of the body from the vagina.

Vagina: A passageway from the cervix to the outside of the body through which the menstruation flows. Although the vaginal walls form a flattened tube at the entrance of which is a fold of tissue called a "hymen" (which may or may not be intact), the vagina can stretch to accommodate a tampon, a penis, and the birth of a baby.

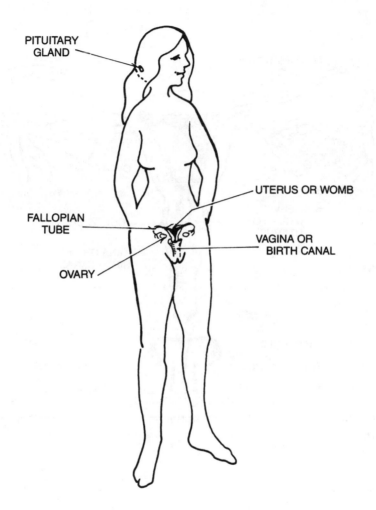

PITUITARY
GLAND

UTERUS OR WOMB

FALLOPIAN
TUBE

VAGINA OR
BIRTH CANAL

OVARY

FEMALE PELVIC ANATOMY

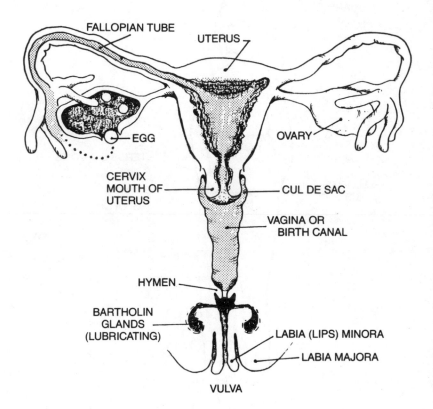

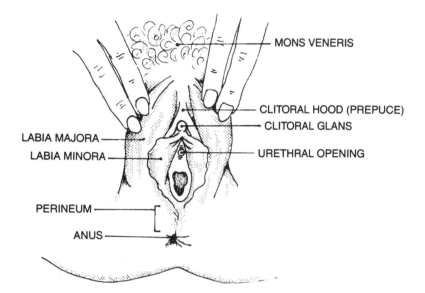

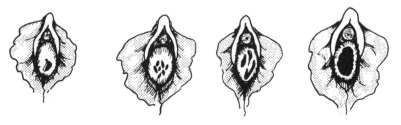

VARIATIONS OF HYMENS

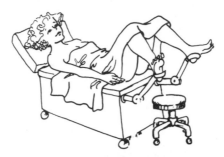

A pelvic exam and a pap test should be performed every year once you become sexually active or have reached the age of 18. The doctor will take your medical history and you may ask questions about your body. After undressing, a gown or sheet is provided for your privacy. As you lie on a table with foot rests (stirrups), the doctor examines the external genitalia and the internal reproductive organs.

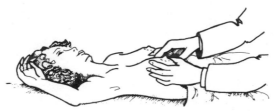

Breast Exam: The doctor examines your breasts while you are sitting and when you are lying down, and will explain how to do a monthly self-breast exam.

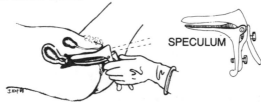

SPECULUM

A Speculum: Available in various sizes, it is a metal or plastic instrument (not sharp) that is gently inserted into the vagina. It holds the vaginal walls apart so the doctor can examine them and the mouth of the uterus (cervix). You may feel pressure from the speculum and it may be cold, but it is not painful.

Pap Smear: A painless test for abnormal cells that may lead to cancer. A blunt wooden stick is used to remove some cells from the cervix and vagina. These are examined under a microscope.

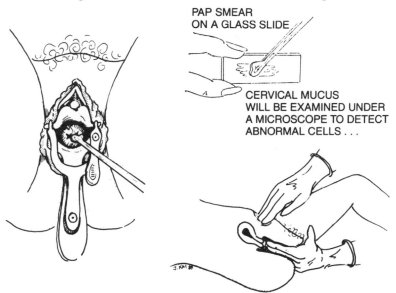

PAP SMEAR
ON A GLASS SLIDE

CERVICAL MUCUS
WILL BE EXAMINED UNDER
A MICROSCOPE TO DETECT
ABNORMAL CELLS . . .

Bi-Manual or Internal Exam: Doctor inserts two fingers into the vagina while gently pressing the abdomen to examine the size and shape of the reproductive organs.

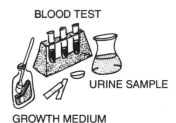

BLOOD TEST

URINE SAMPLE

GROWTH MEDIUM

Other Laboratory Tests: For gonorrhea or herpes culture, fluid from the lesion is taken on a cotton swab and placed in a medium (nutrients) to grow. A blood test for pregnancy, syphilis, and chlamydia, and urine tests for pregnancy and diabetes may be performed. Only after a pelvic exam will the doctor prescribe birth control or medications.

THE MENSTRUAL CYCLE

Day one of the menstrual cycle is the first day of the menstrual flow.
Every woman's cycle is unique. The days below are approximation.

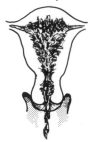

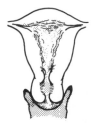

Menstrual Phase:
Days 1–4
The lining of the uterus (endometrium) and the unfertilized egg are shed to create the menstrual flow. Flow continues for 3 to 6 days and contains a tablespoon or two of blood.

Post-Menstrual Phase:
Days 5–8
The ovaries secrete estrogen to thicken the endometrium in readiness to nourish a fertilized egg. In the ovary an egg begins to ripen.

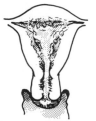

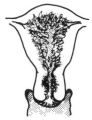

Mid-Menstrual Phase:
Days 9–14
The ovary releases progesterone to enrich the uterine lining. The egg leaves the ovary (ovulation) and travels to the fallopian tube on about the 14th day of the cycle. A woman is at greatest risk of pregnancy during the egg's 4- to 6-day journey through the tube.

Pre-Menstrual Phase:
Days 15–28
Uterine lining continues to grow. If the egg is unfertilized, it disintegrates. Hormone levels drop to trigger menstrual flow, and the lining is shed through the vagina.

MALE REPRODUCTIVE SYSTEM

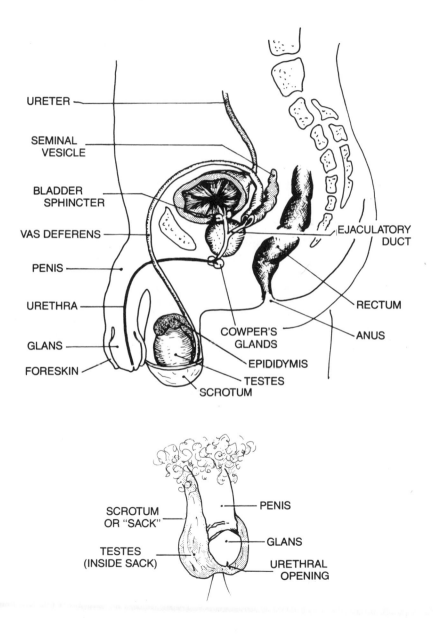

URETER

SEMINAL
VESICLE

BLADDER
SPHINCTER

VAS DEFERENS

PENIS

URETHRA

GLANS

FORESKIN

EJACULATORY
DUCT

RECTUM

ANUS

COWPER'S
GLANDS

EPIDIDYMIS

TESTES

SCROTUM

SCROTUM
OR "SACK"

TESTES
(INSIDE SACK)

PENIS

GLANS

URETHRAL
OPENING

THE EJACULATORY CYCLE

Pituitary Gland: The hypothalamus (at base of the brain) causes the pituitary to release a hormone signaling the testicles to produce sperm.

Scrotum: A loose pouch of skin protecting the testicles from injury and temperature changes.

Testicles or Testes: Throughout a man's life, the testes produce sperm and the hormone testosterone, which regulate male characteristics and sex drive.

Epididymis: Tiny tubules that coil around the testes and store maturing sperm for 2 to 6 weeks.

Vas Deferens: Two long tubes that propel, by muscular contractions, ripened sperm to the seminal vesicle.

Seminal Vesicle: Two glands at the ends of the vas deferens that store sperm and secrete a natural sugar (fructose) to nourish them and add to their mobility as they enter the ejaculatory duct.

Ejaculatory Duct: Two short ducts from either side of the testes passing through the prostate gland.

Prostate Gland: This gland adds a milky substance to the ejaculate to neutralize the acidity of the vagina and the male's urethra, helping to keep sperm alive.

Cowper's Gland: Two glands just below the prostate gland that secret clear droplets at the tip of the penis during sexual excitement. This fluid contains active sperm.

Bladder Sphincter: A small valve at the base of the bladder which closes during sexual arousal to prevent urine from exiting the urethra during ejaculation.

Penis: An organ made up of blood vessels, nerves, and spongy tissue which can become engorged with blood during sexual excitement. It contains no bones.

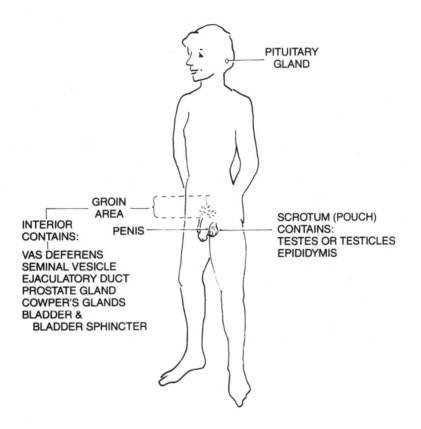

PITUITARY
GLAND

GROIN
AREA

INTERIOR
CONTAINS:

PENIS

VAS DEFERENS
SEMINAL VESICLE
EJACULATORY DUCT
PROSTATE GLAND
COWPER'S GLANDS
BLADDER &
    BLADDER SPHINCTER

SCROTUM (POUCH)
CONTAINS:
TESTES OR TESTICLES
EPIDIDYMIS

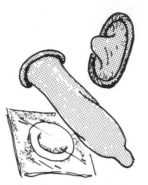

HOW TO PUT ON A CONDOM

Be prepared. Never let erect penis touch vagina, rectum, or mouth of your partner without a condom. The clear fluid released before actual ejaculation contains thousands of sperm and carries the virus that causes AIDS and other sexually transmitted diseases (STDs).

As soon as erection occurs, unroll condom *over the entire penis.* Do not unroll the condom before this time.

Gently press air bubble out of tip (or reservoir) of condom as you unroll it. Air bubbles can interfere with sensitivity and may cause condom to break. This space is needed to catch ejaculate (see illustration).

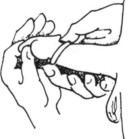

After ejaculating, and *before* penis becomes soft again, withdraw penis and condom together by holding rolled end of condom against base of penis with your fingers to prevent ejaculate from spilling and condom from slipping off inside the vagina (see illustration).

Gently unroll condom from penis and discard in a tissue. Do not allow sex organs to come into contact with partner's genitals after condom is removed.

Condoms should *never* be used more than once.

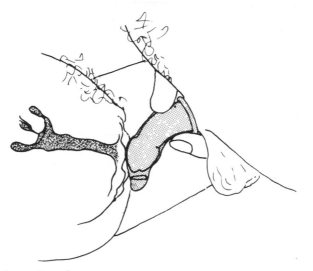

Facts about Condoms

Lambskin or latex: Latex is considered best barrier against AIDS.

Lubricated or dry: Lubricants containing oils (such as Vaseline) *weaken* condoms, and saliva spreads germs. Use water-based lubricants such as K-Y Jelly. Spermicidal lubricants containing the ingredient nonoxynol-9 provide best safeguard against AIDS and STDs. Moist condoms are less likely to break.

Size and shape: Condoms stretch to fit all sizes (circumcised and uncircumcised), but there are size variations. Experiment to find the brand that fits best. Condoms with tip (reservoir) at the end are best for catching ejaculate. Ribbed and ridged condoms may add pleasure for partner. Thickness varies, but is not as important as *age.* Condoms deteriorate after two years and weaken from sun and heat.

Expense: Condoms are inexpensive and are available at all pharmacies.

Effectiveness: Condoms are 95 percent effective when used correctly, with spermicidal foam or jelly (spermicide should contain nonoxynol-9 for best protection against STDs).

Comfort: When condom is tighter at the base, erection lasts longer and orgasm is stronger.

METHOD	WHAT IS IT?	HEALTH CONCERNS
Condoms $1.00–$5.00 (pack of 3)	Also known as "rubbers." Fit over erect penis and catch sperm when the man ejaculates.	Spermicidal condoms containing 0.5 gms of nonoxynol-9 are recommended by AIDS prevention specialists.
Diaphragm $15.00–$16.00 Jelly—$8.00/4 oz.	Rubber cup fits inside vagina, over the opening to the uterus. Used with cream or jelly that kills sperm. Must be fitted by clinician.	Few health problems. More bladder infections for some women. Slight risk of toxic shock syndrome.
Sterilization	Operation that makes a person unable to have a baby. Permanent. Both men and women can be sterilized.	Safer for men than for women. Slight risk of complications after surgery. Tubal pregnancy could occur.
Foam, Suppositories, Cream & Jelly Foam $9.59/1.75 oz. Supp $6.50/12	Chemicals that kill sperm. Put into vagina before intercourse.	None.
IUD (Intrauterine device)	Small device put inside womb by a clinician. Not sure how it works. May stop fertilized egg from implanting and growing in womb.	Increased chance of pelvic inflammatory disease and tubal pregnancy. These 2 problems may impair fertility. Can puncture womb.

STRONG POINTS	WEAK POINTS	EFFECTIVENESS
Highly recommended for "safer sex." Can buy in drugstore. Best protection against sexually transmitted diseases (STDs).	Must be put on during love-making. Some men say it reduces sexual feelings. Condoms with spermicide may irritate vagina or penis.	Used correctly, 2 out of 100 will become pregnant. Used incorrectly, 10 out of 100; used with foam, 1 out of 100.
Can be put in as much as 2 hours before sex. Helps protect against STDs (VD).	Some women say it's hard to insert. Cream or jelly may irritate vagina or penis. Can be messy. Must be left in place 6–8 hours after sex.	Used correctly, 2 out of 100 will become pregnant; used incorrectly, 19 out of 100.
No other contraceptive needed. No effect on sexual desire or ability.	*Permanent.* Cannot change your mind later.	Considered 100 percent.
Can buy in drugstore. Easy to use and carry. Helps protect against STDs (VD).	Must be put in no more than 20 minutes before sex. Can be messy. May irritate vagina or penis.	Used correctly, 3–5 out of 100 will become pregnant. Used incorrectly, 18 out of 100. Used with condoms, 1 out of 100.
Always in place. Doesn't interfere with love-making.	May have more bleeding and cramping during/between periods. Partner may feel IUD string during sex. Should not be used by women with multiple partners.	2–5 out of 100 will become pregnant.

METHOD	WHAT IS IT?	HEALTH CONCERNS
Natural Family Planning	Woman charts several fertility signs—body temperature, vaginal mucus, periods. No intercourse during her fertile time. Special classes needed to learn.	None.
Pill $12–$13/pack (1-month supply)	Pills made of artificial hormones. Stops ovaries from releasing an egg each month. Must be prescribed by a clinician.	Few serious problems for young women. Slight risk of blood clots, heart attacks and strokes. May cause high blood pressure.
Sponge 3/$3.99	Small sponge fits over cervix. Contains chemicals that kill sperm. Sponge blocks or absorbs sperm.	Very small chance of toxic shock syndrome. Should not be used during menstruation. May increase chance of vaginitis.
Withdrawal Coitus Interruptus "Pulling Out" "Russian Roulette"	The penis is withdrawn from the vagina immediately before ejaculation. Ejaculation occurs completely away from the vagina and the external genitalia of the female.	May cause emotional stress because of the need to pull out in time.

STRONG POINTS	WEAK POINTS	EFFECTIVENESS
Acceptable to most religious beliefs.	Must chart *every day*. No sex during fertile time. If periods aren't regular, may not be as effective.	Used correctly, 2–20 out of 100 will become pregnant; used incorrectly, 20–25 out of 100 will become pregnant.
Simple and easy to use. Doesn't interfere with love-making. Less bleeding and cramping during period.	Possible weight changes, moodiness, spotting. Must take every day. Not advisable for women over 35.	Used correctly, 1 out of 100 will become pregnant. Used incorrectly, 2 out of 100 will become pregnant.
Can buy in drugstore. Can be put in several hours before love-making and left in up to 24 hours. Helps protect against STDs.	Sponge can tear during removal. May irritate vagina or penis. May not be as effective for women who have had children. May cause vaginal dryness.	Used correctly, 11–19 out of 100 will become pregnant; used incorrectly, 10–20 out of 100 will become pregnant.
Requires no devices or chemicals. No cost.	Semen often escapes from penis before ejaculation. One drop contains millions of sperm. May diminish sexual pleasure for a couple.	Highest failure rate of all birth control methods. 16–23 pregnancies per 100 women among active users.

*

Index